# AT THE FRONT LINES OF MEDICINE

# AT THE FRONT LINES OF MEDICINE

How the Health Care System Alienates
Doctors and Mistreats Patients . . .
and What We Can Do about It

## HOWARD WAITZKIN

ROWMAN & LITTLEFIELD PUBLISHERS, INC.
*Lanham • Boulder • New York • Oxford*

ROWMAN & LITTLEFIELD PUBLISHERS, INC.

Published in the United States of America
by Rowman & Littlefield Publishers, Inc.
4720 Boston Way, Lanham, Maryland 20706
www.rowmanlittlefield.com

12 Hid's Copse Road
Cumnor Hill, Oxford OX2 9JJ, England

British Library Cataloguing in Publication Information Available

**Library of Congress Cataloging-in-Publication Data**

Waitzkin, Howard.
    At the front lines of medicine : how the health care system alienates doctors
and mistreats patients . . . and what we can do about it / Howard Waitzkin.
        p. cm.
    Includes bibliographical references and index.
    ISBN 0-7425-0131-0 (alk. paper)
        1. Social medicine—United States. 2. Medical care—Social aspects—
United States. 3. Health services accessibility—United States. 4. Poor—
Medical care—United States. I. Title.
    RA418.3.U6 W35 2001
    362.1′0973—dc21

                                                                2001019739

Printed in the United States of America

**Copyright acknowledgment**

The author and publisher gratefully acknowledge permission to use the
quoted material from *Waiting for Lefty* by Clifford Odets. Copyright © 1993
by Grove/Atlantic, Inc.

*For the many* FRIENDS AND COLLEAGUES *who have struggled
in the practice of social medicine in Latin America,*

*and for* JOHN STOECKLE,
*primary care practitioner, mentor, and social critic.*

*They have struggled for a just society as the necessary context
for the humane and effective practice of medicine.*

BARNES   So they told you?

BENJ   Told me what?

BARNES   They're closing Ward C next month. I don't have to tell you the hospital isn't self supporting. Until last year that board of trustees met deficits. . . . You can guess the rest. At a board meeting Tuesday, our fine feathered friends discovered they couldn't meet the last quarter's deficit—a neat little sum well over $100,000. If the hospital is to continue at all, it's damn—

BENJ   Necessary to close another charity ward!

BARNES   So they say . . .

\*   \*   \*

BARNES   Doctors don't run medicine in this country. The men who know their jobs don't run anything here, except motormen on trolley cars. I've seen medicine change—plenty—anesthesia, sterilization—but not because of rich men—in *spite* of them! In a rich man's country your true self's buried deep. . . .

\*   \*   \*

BENJ   Last week I was thinking about it—the wonderful opportunity to work in their socialized medicine.

BARNES   Beautiful, beautiful!

BENJ   Nothing's nearer what I'd like to do!

BARNES   Do it!

BENJ   No! Our work's here—America! I'm scared. . . . What future's ahead, I don't know.

—**Clifford Odets, *Waiting for Lefty*, 1935**
**("Interne Episode")**

# contents

◆ ◆

ix

# preface

◆ ◆

This book grew from personal experiences that shaped my perceptions about health and society. My family struggled with poverty. Throughout my childhood and adolescence, my parents, both office workers, dealt with unstable employment and feared illness partly because of its financial impact. Several members of my family suffered from financial barriers to health care services, as they either delayed or did without care that they felt they needed.

These barriers even affected me. When I was thirteen, I broke my right leg sliding into third base. Because of spotty follow-up care while my leg was in a cast, I was left with a difference in leg length that eventually led to scoliosis of the spine and neurologic effects. During the summer before my fifteenth birthday, when my parents told me I needed to support myself, I got a job selling encyclopedias door-to-door, which allowed me to stay in school and even save some money for college. Of course, this job did not include health insurance, so I continued to lack follow-up care for my orthopedic problem.

Beyond their impact on my understanding, personal experiences also influenced my commitments to change. My parents' financial problems included the loss of the first and only home that they were able to buy. This loss resulted from blockbusting real-estate tactics, where homeowners were pressured to sell their homes cheaply in response to rumors that an influx of black neighbors would reduce property values. When we moved, I had to leave several black friends in the neighborhood. In high school, I got involved in struggles about civil rights and access to public services. As a crusading high-school newspaper editor, I organized a successful boycott of local barbershops that refused to cut the hair of black students; along the way, I had to deal emotionally with a handwritten death threat from the Ku Klux Klan of northeastern Ohio.

My grandfather, a farmer who lost his land during the Depression and who later became a house painter and union organizer, influenced my views on social justice. With gentle humor and fierce courage in his piercing green eyes, he taught me early on about his organizing efforts in support of Eugene Debs's populist presidential campaigns, as well as the struggle to form unions in Akron, home of the first industrial sit-ins. When I was sixteen, he died from liver cancer, which probably resulted from exposure to organic solvents used in painting. The devastating process of his dying, in which doctors and family members tried to keep the truth from him to help preserve his morale, led me to pursue a career in medicine, but with a different path from those taken by doctors I had met.

My work in medicine has taken place in several primary care settings, usually based in communities where many of my patients and coworkers have come from low-income and minority backgrounds. I have focused on improving access to needed services and on social problems that affect the process and outcomes of care. In addition to clinical work in community clinics and public hospitals, I have tried to conduct action-oriented research and take part in primary care teaching.

These efforts have taken place mainly in three settings. Between 1978 and 1982, after finishing my residency in internal medicine at Massachusetts General Hospital, I worked as a primary care internist at La Clínica de la Raza, a community health center in Oakland, California. There we tried to respond to the needs of a large, underserved population of working people and immigrants, both documented and undocumented. During this period, I also did clinical teaching with medical students from the University of California, San Francisco, and taught public health and sociology at the University of California, Berkeley.

In 1982, I accepted a job as professor and director of general internal medicine and primary care at the University of California, Irvine. Through this role, I tried to foster primary care training and clinical efforts, mainly at a university-affiliated community health center in an underserved area of Orange County. Due to the unsupportive public policies of the county government, as well as cutbacks in public funding at the state and federal levels, I became involved in a series of difficult struggles aimed at reducing access barriers. These struggles also required research that demonstrated the widespread problems people faced locally in obtaining needed services.

In 1997, I moved to the University of New Mexico as professor and director of community medicine. There I have worked with a public health program that collaborates with students and communities throughout the Southwest region. Many of these communities are characterized by poverty, geographic isolation, and cultural marginalization, all of which exert adverse effects on health and mental health outcomes. In New Mexico I also have continued my work as a primary care internist at the university hospital, which attempts to serve a large, multicultural community, including many patients who suffer from poverty and barriers to access.

In all these efforts as a health care worker, teacher, and researcher, I have experienced on a personal level the agonizing crisis of access and costs, which has grown ever deeper during the 1980s and 1990s, and now in the new millennium. I also have participated in national and local efforts to construct a more responsive health care system. These work experiences have added to those that earlier affected my family and myself. All these experiences have contributed to my chronic outrage about health care in the United States and have deepened my quest with many others to seek fundamental change. Such change must occur not only in the health care system, but also in the broader society that shapes health services and fundamentally affects the health of our population.

In the United States, such realizations seem to recur with each generation. That is my point in framing this book, at the beginning and end, with the outrage and optimism of Dr. Benjamin, the impassioned medical resident of Clifford Odets's play, *Waiting for Lefty*. This play appeared more than sixty years ago, yet it conveys much the same message as I am trying to communicate now. All other economically developed countries have acted decisively to overcome these problems. Enough decades have passed, the problems and potential solutions are not mysterious, and further delay only deepens the suffering in our midst.

This book developed from such practical work "at the front lines" of medicine. I aim to describe some of the most important problems that face us today, point out directions of progressive change, describe the impediments that stand in the way of change, and discuss how these impediments can be overcome.

Throughout the book, I argue that problems of health care are closely linked to problems of society. From this viewpoint, a just health care system—a system that responds in a humane and ethical way to human needs—is also linked to the achievement of a more just society. At the start of a new millennium, barriers to access and the enormous costs of care in the United States have become ever more intolerable, except to those who profit from the current unjust arrangements. These structural conditions of the health care system injure our dignity as individuals and the dignity of our society.

The correction of these problems, which would bring the United States at least into the company of other economically advantaged countries, requires not only reforms in health policy, but also changes in the broader society, especially in social hierarchies based on class, race, gender, and age. I argue that local efforts in communities can lead to important changes, but that these changes have to build toward a national health program that guarantees universal access to needed care. Yet, although accessible and affordable medical care can address many important needs, overall outcomes such as mortality and survival for specific diseases depend much more on individuals' social class positions and race than on the medical care that they do or do not receive. For that reason, proposals for a national health program in the United States also must be linked to struggles aimed at changing the oppressive social structures that lead to illness and early death.

Here are some comments on the book's organization and main themes.

Part one links concrete clinical problems with social policy issues that hinder primary care. In the first chapter, I present the case histories of actual patients who illustrate different types of barriers to health care access, and then move from these clinical presentations to the national problems of access and costs. This chapter also documents the failure of previous policies in addressing these national problems. Chapter two examines the gap between knowledge about problems and the power to solve them. In exploring this issue, I focus especially on the relationship between local problems and global policies intended as solutions. Chapter three, which analyzes the social origins of illness and early death, questions whether changes in health policy can address some of the most fundamental health problems that confront us.

In part two, I deal with the ways that social problems impinge on the primary care encounter, again with a perspective that links this encounter to the broader social context in which it takes place. Chapter four describes the changes in the relationships between patients and doctors, and especially changes in communication, that have occurred in the era of managed care. Mental health problems that arise in primary care—depression; abuse; situational reactions to job loss, homelessness, and financial stress; trauma associated with violence and migration; and unexplained somatic symptoms among immigrants and refugees—are the focus of chapter five.

Part three looks at proposed solutions, especially the strengths and weaknesses of national and local proposals for improved health care access and reduced costs. In chapter six, I describe local struggles for access and control of health institutions, including advocacy for the "medically indigent" and resistance against corporate takeover of hospitals and clinics. Chapter seven analyzes the two major options most recently considered as models for a national health program in the United States: managed care versus a "single-payer" system. Then, chapter eight discusses problems that would not be solved simply through a national health program—especially patterns of mortality and adverse health outcomes that are closely linked to structures of inequality based on social class, race, and gender; the chapter discusses an agenda for wider social changes as the basis for improved health outcomes. In conclusion, chapter nine proposes solutions at the level of the patient–doctor relationship; these proposals include a more direct approach to social problems that arise in primary care encounters and a response to mental health problems in primary care that encourages cultural sensitivity and empowerment.

# acknowledgments

◆ ◆

In this work, I have been fortunate to receive feedback, emotional support, inspiration, role modeling, and love, as well as some very helpful financial support, from many friends and coworkers. I'd like to acknowledge some of them here.

*In Physicians for a National Health Program:* Tom Bodenheimer, Ken Frisof, Kevin Grumbach, David Himmelstein, Ida Hellender, Norty Kalishman, Bruce Trigg, Steffie Woolhandler, and Quentin Young.

*In Latin America:* Jaime Breilh, Marcos Buchbinder, Arturo Campaña, José Carlos Escudero, Alfredo Estrada, Celia Iriart, Cristina Laurell, Francisco Mercado, Emerson Elias Merhy, Francisco Rojas Ochoa, Jaime Sepúlveda, Mario Testa, Carolina Tetelboin, and Adriana Vega.

*At the University of New Mexico, Health Centers of Northern New Mexico, and New Mexico Department of Health:* Dave Coultas, Marilyn Diener, Bonnie Duran, Jo Fairbanks, Joe Gallegos, Deborah Helitzer, Norty Kalishman, Louise Lamphere, Carolyn Lara-Smith, Rae Lewis, Gloria López, Lorraine Halinka Malcoe, Gaye Martínez, Richard Santos, Saverio Sava, Terry Schleder, David Stolze, Mark Unverzagt, Frances Varela, Nina Wallerstein, Allene Whitney, Bill Wiese, Rob Williams, and Joel Yager.

xvii

(Terry Schleder, Rae Lewis, and Allene Whitney provided very helpful research assistance for this book.)

*At the Agency for Healthcare Research and Quality:* Carolyn Clancy, Jayasree Basu, and Skip Moyer (who facilitated grant 1R01 HS09703).

*At the Fogarty International Center of the National Institutes of Health:* Mirilee Pearl and Heidi Schwab (who facilitated grant TW01982).

*At the National Institute of Mental Health:* Ann Hohmann, Kenneth Lutterman, and Junius Gonzales (who facilitated grants 1R01 MH47536, 1R24 MH58404, and 1R25 MH60288).

*At the National Library of Medicine:* Frances Johnson (who facilitated grant 1G08 LM06688).

*At Rowman & Littlefield:* Dean Birkenkamp.

I also gratefully acknowledge the contributions of David Himmelstein, Steffie Woolhandler, Vicente Navarro, and Physicians for a National Health Program for the preparation of the figures that appear in chapters one and seven.

# ◆ part one ◆

## PRIMARY CARE AND SOCIAL POLICY

# ◆ chapter one ◆

# Access, Costs, and the Failure of Past Policies

## THE HUMAN EXPERIENCE OF ACCESS BARRIERS

Barriers to health care access have become pervasive in the United States. These barriers prevent patients from receiving needed services but also impose fundamental ethical problems for doctors and other health workers who find themselves unable to solve problems that sometimes lead to patients' deaths and continuing disabilities. As I describe in the preface, I have tried to deal with these barriers throughout most of my career in medicine. I have shared with patients, students, and colleagues the anguish of not being able to receive or to provide needed services, due to the lack of suitable public policies.

The following summaries depict the experiences of patients I have seen personally, or who have been seen by faculty members, residents, and students with whom I have worked at community clinics. Although they do not depict comprehensively all the barriers to access that patients experience in the United States, these stories give a human face to the troubling statistical data on access barriers, which I then describe. The stories also will give a context for the policy analyses and recommendations for change that follow in later chapters.

3

## U.S. Citizens Suffering from Cutbacks and Increased Copayments under Medicaid

The first two patients illustrate problems of access for patients covered under Medicaid, the national program that aims to assure access to care for eligible, low-income people. Medicaid covers individuals with dependent children, those who are disabled, and many people in nursing homes. To be eligible, a person must earn a monthly income that falls below the level of poverty as determined by the state and federal governments.

*A 31-year-old diabetic and legally blind man began to experience severe unilateral headaches but could not afford a computerized tomographic (CT) scan of the head because his monthly deductible under Medicaid, which he was required to pay out of pocket each month, increased from $50 to $250. He later was brought delirious to the emergency room, where an emergency CT scan revealed a brain tumor with poor prognosis. At his death, his physicians felt that the tumor may have been resected successfully if he had received attention earlier, when his severe headaches first began.*

*A 56-year-old man with metastatic soft-tissue sarcoma could not afford follow-up visits, medications, visiting nurse, or hospice because his deductible under Medicaid had increased to $350 per month. This patient died in pain and without adequate nursing support in his home because of financial barriers.*

## U.S. Citizens Facing Restrictions Due to Policies of a County-Administered Medically Indigent Adult (MIA) Program

The next group of patients could not receive needed care despite their eligibility for medical benefits under the county government's program for MIAs. This program covers adults who are not eligible for federal Medicaid but whose income is below the state-defined poverty limit. To reduce costs, many states decentralized MIA programs to county governments during the early 1980s. Counties vary widely in services provided and in copayments required from patients.

*A 63-year-old man with hypertension, renal insufficiency, and prostatic enlargement causing urinary obstruction could not gain approval from*

*the county's MIA program for a prostatectomy, because it was consid-*
*ered an elective procedure. His urinary obstruction and renal function*
*gradually worsened. When he finally required dialysis, he became eligi-*
*ble for federal Medicare benefits. The massive costs of dialysis (more*
*than $100,000 per year) could have been avoided if he had received a*
*prostatectomy initially.*

*A 29-year-old woman presented with a breast mass. Mammography*
*was consistent with cancer. Approval of MIA funding for outpatient*
*biopsy was delayed for more than a month during the eligibility screen-*
*ing process because the condition was not considered an emergency. At*
*the time of surgery, the cancer had not metastasized to her lymph*
*nodes, but the patient and her physicians remained worried that the*
*delay, which was much longer than typically experienced by an insured*
*woman with a breast mass, may have jeopardized her prognosis.*

*A 44-year-old man had malignant melanoma, confirmed by limited*
*biopsy with incomplete excision. Outpatient surgery for wider resection*
*was delayed for more than three months by MIA eligibility procedures,*
*again because the procedure was considered elective. By the time that*
*the biopsy was performed, the melanoma had metastasized widely, and*
*the patient subsequently died.*

*A 52-year-old man developed unstable angina after a myocardial infarc-*
*tion. The MIA program disapproved funding for elective coronary*
*angiography, even though national standards of cardiologic practice*
*required its being performed under these circumstances.*

### People Whose Physicians Abandon Them Because of Inability to Pay

Many patients in the United States have established relationships with physicians who follow them for many years
until they lose their insurance, because of job loss, a company's
decision not to provide insurance as a fringe benefit, divorce or
death of a spouse, geographic relocation, or other changes in
circumstances. At the time that the patients lose their insurance, doctors frequently decline to follow them because of perceived barriers that prevent the patient from paying full fees.
"Abandonment" is a legal principle by which a doctor is prevented from declining to see a patient whom the doctor previously has followed, unless a suitable substitute is arranged and
the patient agrees to this arrangement.[1] Nevertheless, neither

governmental agencies nor professional organizations enforce these principles in cases when patients lose insurance.

*The 63-year-old man with hypertension, renal insufficiency, and prostatic enlargement causing urinary obstruction, described above, had worked for many years as a custodian for a small health maintenance organization (HMO). While he worked there, one of the HMO's physicians saw him informally for his high blood pressure. Because the HMO did not provide health care as a fringe benefit for its own nonprofessional employees, these visits generally were provided as a free service by the physician, who believed that an employee with a major health problem should receive at least some needed care. After a cutback, however, the HMO laid off this patient from his job, and the physician decided that he no longer could justify offering free services. As a result, the patient spent several months with inadequate blood-pressure control, until he could be seen at a local community clinic.*

*A 44-year-old unemployed woman was followed by her physician for about eight years because of reflex sympathetic dystrophy, a very painful condition of her legs and feet that periodically required low doses of a narcotic and a tranquilizer for symptom relief. When the patient went through a divorce, she lost her husband's insurance coverage. Shortly thereafter, her long-term physician informed her that he could no longer see her because she lacked insurance. Several months passed, during which she could not receive needed treatment, until a physician at a community clinic agreed to see her.*

### People Who Delay Treatment for Cancer Due to Lack of Insurance and Therefore Die Unnecessarily from Metastatic Disease

One of the most troubling effects of access barriers in the United States involves preventable deaths that could be avoided if people could obtain the care that they need. In our experience, such tragedies arise most commonly when patients cannot find appropriate services for the diagnosis and treatment of cancer. When symptoms of cancer arise, such patients experience critical delays, with a deleterious impact on the eventual outcome of their disease. Problems in cancer services arise for patients who face access barriers despite coverage by public insurance, as noted previously. Barriers become especially grim, however, when patients lack insurance altogether.

*A 48-year-old Japanese-American woman ran her own small landscape-gardening business. Because of the high cost of individual health-insurance policies, she decided to remain uninsured. After noticing a breast lump, she delayed seeking care because she did not have a regular doctor and because she feared the expenses of care; she hoped the mass would disappear. When the mass continued to grow after three months, she began to seek care from private physicians, who declined to see her due to lack of insurance. After six months, she eventually was able to find care at a community clinic. Evaluation for metastatic disease was arranged by special request with a nuclear medicine facility at a university hospital; without the personal intervention of her physicians and the donation of specialty services, the appropriate scan would not have been done. The scan revealed extensive metastatic cancer. Her chemotherapy also was delayed because of access barriers. Within six months, the patient died.*

### Homeless People's Lack of Housing That Inhibits Effective Treatment of Serious Medical Problems

Other social problems in U.S. society heighten the impact of barriers to health care access; among these problems, one of the most important is homelessness, which inhibits effective treatment of serious medical problems, including infectious diseases like tuberculosis that threaten the health of the general community. Despite their poverty, homeless people experience difficulty in obtaining needed care under public insurance programs. For instance, many programs require an address to assure that the expenses of care are assigned to the correct county or other governmental unit. Because they cannot provide an address, homeless people frequently cannot obtain public coverage. In addition, they tend to be more vulnerable to access barriers even when covered.

*A 52-year-old homeless man fell and fractured his hip. Although he could not walk, he struggled to hitch rides to the emergency rooms of two nearby private hospitals. Because he was uninsured and unkempt, and because his problem did not appear life-threatening, the triage personnel at these emergency rooms advised the patient that he could not be seen without a large cash deposit. The next day, he was picked up by police after he was found crawling along a curb and was taken to a local community clinic, where the fractured hip was diagnosed. Despite his lack of insurance coverage, he was admitted to a university hospital for surgery.*

*A 38-year-old uninsured, homeless man was admitted to a university
hospital from the emergency room because of active pulmonary tuberculosis. He had come to the emergency room because he was coughing up
blood. During a week of hospitalization, he was treated with three
antibiotics, until his sputum was free of organisms. Due to financial
problems, the hospital recently had initiated a policy that outpatient
prescriptions would not be filled unless they were paid for directly by
the patient or were chargeable to public or private insurance. For this
reason, the patient was asked to travel after discharge to the county
health department for his outpatient prescriptions to continue necessary
treatment for tuberculosis. However, the patient did not find transportation and consequently did not receive his outpatient medications.
Four weeks later, he again developed bloody sputum and was readmitted
for active tuberculosis; this time, his treatment became more complicated since he had developed a medication-resistant organism because of
the interruption in antibiotics.*

## Undocumented Immigrants

Undocumented immigrants are another important group of
patients experiencing major barriers to access, as they are not
covered under most public programs. Such immigrants contribute substantially to the economic productivity of the United
States, especially in the Southwest and Southeast regions, and
pay much more in taxes than they receive in public benefits.[2]
Although they tend to be healthier and utilize health care services less than age-matched U.S. citizens,[3] they have few options
for care when illness strikes.

*A 22-year-old woman from Costa Rica, without legal documents, pre-
sented with cardiac enlargement and a right axillary mass. For two
months, arrangements could not be made for an echo-cardiogram or
biopsy of the mass. As a result, the patient moved to another county
in California with less restrictive policies about medical care for the
undocumented.*

*A 31-year-old undocumented man from Mexico presented with carpal
tunnel syndrome of his right hand that interfered with his work as a
tailor. He had worked and had taxes deducted from his pay at a local
clothing factory for the past 18 years. Acromegaly associated with a
pituitary tumor was diagnosed, but radiation therapy or neurosurgery
could not be arranged because of financial impediments. After waiting*

*nearly three months, the patient was lost to follow-up when he returned to Mexico.*

### People Who Have Lost Insurance Due to Job Loss

The following two cases show the special problems of working people who lose their insurance because of job loss. They also illustrate issues that I have found especially important for the work in health-services research and policy that I describe later.

*A 55-year-old man who served as an office worker in a small horticultural company lost his job after 25 years with that firm. One month later, he lost his health insurance, which had been provided as a fringe benefit of employment. After another month, he suddenly passed out and was taken to a county hospital because his private physician refused to see him without insurance. He was diagnosed with upper gastrointestinal hemorrhage from a bleeding duodenal ulcer, with resulting loss of consciousness. After treatment with transfusions and medications, the patient slowly recovered. Nearly one year after losing his job, the patient found employment again as an office worker, received insurance coverage, and returned to his former physician for care.*

*A 53-year-old receptionist and clerical worker was not working, partly because of symptoms of pain and limited mobility associated with premature osteoporosis. She relied on the insurance coverage of her husband, the patient in the previous case summary. About three months after he lost his job, she fell and fractured her forearm and wrist. Her private physician would not see her without insurance coverage. She was taken to the county hospital, where resident physicians tried to realign the fractures, but she was left with a deformity.*

These two patients have influenced my commitments in primary care and health policy, because they are my own parents. My father and mother experienced these problems just as I was completing my residency training in internal medicine. They are proud people, who have worked hard throughout their lives and have been very reluctant to avail themselves of public welfare or insurance programs. They asked me not to intercede with their physicians or the hospital staff where they were taken, since they viewed their problems as their own responsibility. At various times, they expressed the view that they somehow deserved the misfortunes that have befallen them, because they had not found a way to attend college during and after the Great Depression.

My parents' experiences illustrate two central themes regarding barriers to health care access in the United States. First, these barriers involve fundamental issues of personal dignity. The difficulties faced by my parents and the other patients described above degrade the individuals and families involved, at a time when they are most in need. Personal dignity requires more from social policy than we have yet achieved in the United States.

Second, such problems can happen to anyone, largely as a matter of luck. Severe illness can strike people who have lived their lives in accord with the mainstream standards of their communities. When misfortune arises, the United States does not provide a "safety net" that assures access to basic medical services. Further, these problems do not affect only poor people and members of minority groups, although their impact is particular severe for such individuals and families. Instead, barriers to access can exert unpredictable and devastating effects for a large part of the U.S. population, including a substantial part of the middle class.

## THE NATIONAL PROBLEMS OF ACCESS AND COSTS

Having described barriers to access at the level of individual, flesh-and-blood patients who suffer from these problems, I now turn to the national level. The United States remains the only economically developed country in the world without a national health program that assures universal access to basic health care services. Barriers to access and escalating costs of care have created a chronic crisis, which will continue as a target of policy during coming years.

### Access

At the beginning of the twenty-first century, more than 43 million people in the United States lacked health insurance. This number, representing approximately 14 percent of the population, has increased by about 10 million persons during the past decade. Most of the uninsured are working people

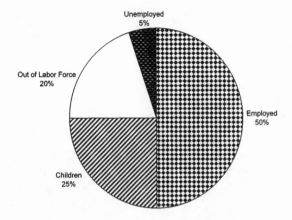

**FIGURE 1.1** *Who are the uninsured in the United States? (Out of labor force: students older than 18, homemakers, the disabled, early retirees.)*
Source: Himmelstein and Woolhandler, tabulation from 1999 CPS.

(figure 1.1). Uninsured workers are spread across company size, as both large and small businesses frequently do not pay for health insurance as a fringe benefit of employment.

In addition to the uninsured, approximately 50 million people are underinsured. These are persons who, even though they hold health insurance policies, would be bankrupted by a major illness, which is currently the most frequent cause of personal bankruptcy in the United States. The underinsured include many elderly people, as well as a substantial part of the so-called middle class. For instance, Medicare pays for less than half of the medical expenses of senior citizens over 65 years of age, and elderly people spend more money out-of-pocket on health care, in inflation-controlled dollars, than they did before the enactment of Medicare in 1965. More than five million young women hold insurance policies that exclude maternity care. Many more millions of people cannot use their insurance because of copayments, deductibles, exclusions, or preexisting medical conditions that disqualify them from coverage. U.S. private insurance ironically excludes those who need it most: people with preexisting illness.

Public programs do not adequately protect people who experience such barriers. For example, the national Medicaid pro-

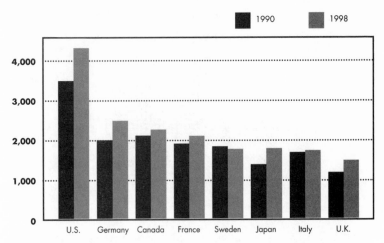

**FIGURE 1.2** *Comparative international health spending, 1990 and 1998, 1998 U.S. dollars, adjusted for purchasing power parity.*
Source: Health Affairs (19[3], 2000: 150).

gram, which was initiated to provide needed care for poor people, has proven insufficient and has deteriorated over time. States have varied widely in the proportion of the population below the poverty level who are covered by Medicaid, and on the average the proportion of the poverty population eligible for Medicaid benefits has declined markedly since 1980.

## Costs

In spite of these terrible problems of access, the costs of health care in the United States have continued to grow. Uncontrolled costs thus have become the second major part of the nation's health crisis. In 1999, these costs totaled more than $1 trillion annual, or about 14 percent of the gross domestic product. Between 1985 and 1992, health spending nearly doubled, despite explicit policies to control costs, including the expansion of managed care, the initiation of Medicare's program of diagnosis-related groups, and the spread of mandated utilization review. Although costs to corporations that purchased health insurance for employees moderated during the mid-1990s, these costs began to increase again during the late 1990s; costs to consumers continued to increase during the entire decade, as corporate employers passed on a greater proportion of their costs to employees.[4]

The costs of health care in the United States far exceed those of any other country. For instance, on both an absolute and per capita basis, the United States spends much more on health care than any of the economically developed nations of Europe, Canada, and Japan. All these other countries, despite their lower health care costs, have initiated national health programs that provide universal access to needed services. Figure 1.2 shows these cross-national comparisons as of the late 1990s.

Although uncontrolled costs constitute a multifaceted problem, administrative waste deserves special emphasis.[5] Figure 1.3 shows the growth of physicians and administrators in the U.S. health care system since 1970. As can be seen, administrators represent the fastest-growing sector of the health care labor force, expanding at three times the rate of physicians and other clinical personnel. The United States spends more than any other economically developed country on administration, which consumes approximately 25 percent of health care costs. This figure compares unfavorably to all countries with national health programs, which spend between 6 and 18 percent of

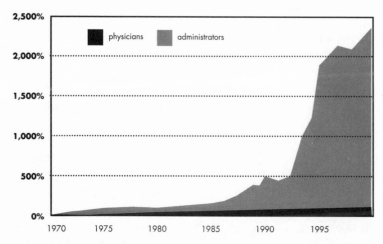

**FIGURE 1.3** *Growth of physicians and administrators, 1970–1998.*
Source: Bureau of Labor Statistics and NCHS.

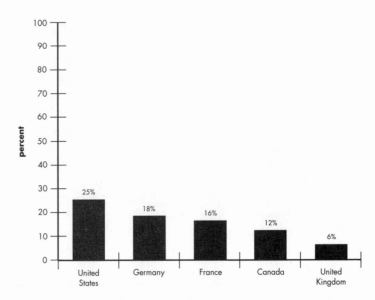

**FIGURE 1.4** *Administrative expenses as a percentage of all health care expenses.*

health care costs on administration (figure 1.4). If the United States could reduce administrative spending to a proportion comparable to that of countries with national health programs, the savings (currently about 10 percent of total expenditures of $1 trillion, or about $100 billion) would be adequate to provide universal access to health services without additional spending.[6]

How might administrative savings be achieved to help control costs? To answer this question, let me discuss the nurse shown in figure 1.5. As judged by the spots on her uniform, this nurse suffers from a common hospital-acquired infection, "billing-sticker-itis." These stickers come from the sources shown in figure 1.6. In most U.S. hospitals, each intravenous line, each medication, each gown, each surgical instrument, and each toothbrush has a billing sticker attached to it. A typical nurse like this one spends between 10 and 30 percent of her or his time on gathering together these stickers and related administrative functions. The billing stickers are converted to cards or other pieces of paper and sent to the hospital's billing depart-

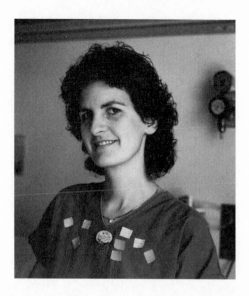

**FIGURE 1.5** *A nurse suffering from hospital-acquired infection.*

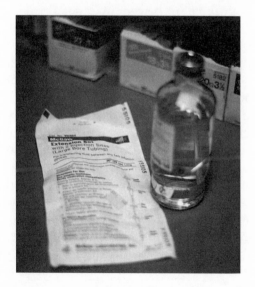

**FIGURE 1.6** *Source of the nurse's hospital-acquired infection, "billing-sticker-itis."*

ment, where, in a typical urban hospital, more than a hundred employees computerize the charges and prepare separate bills for the more than a thousand insurance companies that process private and public insurance claims. These companies differ widely in their reporting requirements, billing procedures, copayments, deductibles, exclusions, and other policies. Such different provisions greatly increase the administrative costs of submitting bills by hospitals and practitioners.

A national health program in the United States could drastically reduce such wasteful administrative practices by eliminating the need for billing in hospitals. As in Canada and several European countries, hospitals could be funded through global annual budgets negotiated with the national health program, rather than the present costly and cumbersome billing apparatus. From the standpoint of insurance companies, administrative overhead is a rapidly growing component of costs. Overall, insurance overhead has increased to represent nearly 1 percent of the gross domestic product of the United States, compared with about 0.1 percent in Canada.

An additional component of administrative waste arises from the intense marketing and advertising of medical products. U.S. pharmaceutical and supply firms annually spend more than $10 billion on advertising and "detailing" of drugs and other medical products; this figure exceeds the total costs for teaching medical students in the United States. Such promotional activities are intended to influence physicians' prescribing habits. Patients and/or insurers bear the costs of these promotional activities through higher than necessary drug prices. Again, such wasteful practices could be restricted under a national health program that would provide needed medications and supplies but at a lower overall cost.

In summary, we face a cruel contradiction in the United States. On the one hand, at least a third of our population face barriers to health care access because of lack of insurance, underinsurance, or insurance that cannot be used to meet existing needs. On the other hand, we spend more money on health care than any other nation, and the costs of care continue to rise at a rate that threatens our economic security. Paradoxically, the numbers of uninsured in the United States have increased roughly in parallel to increases in spending.

## THE FAILURE OF PAST POLICIES

At the heart of the health policy debate in the United States has been the question of health care as a basic human right. On the individual level is the issue of the inherent value of each person, and whether that value then entitles one to health care. The concept of a right to needed services is not new to this country; for instance, the constitutional right to legal representation guarantees that all individuals are entitled to basic services. However, the U.S. Constitution does not provide for a clear right to health care, in contrast to the constitutions of many other countries.[7]

### Policy Options

*Competitive strategies.* Since the 1980s, competitive strategies have achieved prominence in health policy circles. Such proposals aim to foster competition among providers and thus lower costs.[8] Competitive strategies culminated in "managed competition," a policy option favored initially by the Clinton administration. The basic assumption is that by allowing competitive forces of the market to control health care delivery, competitive policies would result in a high-quality, cost-effective system.

Competitive strategies have received major criticism. Forces of competition generally have not controlled health care costs, as illustrated by the rise in overall costs at a rate higher than general inflation and by higher costs in regions with greater competition among health care providers.[9] Further, medical services never have shown the characteristics of a competitive market, since government pays for more than 40 percent of health care and since the insurance, pharmaceutical, and medical equipment industries all manifest monopolistic tendencies that inhibit competition. Hospitals and physicians maintain political-economic power through professional organizations that reduce the impact of competitive strategies. Physicians also affect the demand for services through recommendations about referrals, diagnostic studies, and treatment. Analytically, the effects of competition on costs are difficult to separate from other important changes, especially the effects of general inflation, the requirement of major copayments by patients, and the impact of mandatory prepayment. Additionally, competitive strategies do not curtail administrative waste.

Such competitive strategies in public programs also have led to major dislocations and gaps in services.[10] For example, competitive contracting and prospective reimbursement under Medicaid have worsened the financial crises of hospitals with a large proportion of indigent clients. The resultant disruption in services due to underfunding of Medicaid has led to a measurable worsening of some patients' medical conditions. In some states, competitive health plans have suffered severe and unpredicted financial problems, and patients have encountered major barriers to access, including direct refusal of care by providers.

Several ethical issues also have arisen with competitive strategies. On an individual level, autonomy may be compromised through elimination of a consumer's free choice of physicians and hospitals. Increased out-of-pocket costs may further impair autonomy by restricting access to care, especially among the poor. A two-tiered system remains in place, as the working poor and unemployed receive more limited coverage than the wealthy.

*Corporate involvement in health care.* Various policies have encouraged corporate expansion in the medical field. By the mid-1970s, private insurance companies, pharmaceutical firms, and medical equipment manufacturers already had achieved prominent positions in the medical marketplace. In the 1980s and 1990s, multinational corporations took over community hospitals in all regions of the country, acquired and/or managed many public hospitals, bought or built teaching hospitals affiliated with medical schools, and gained control of ambulatory care organizations.[11]

Corporate profitability in health care has encountered few obstacles, despite declines in profit margins for some corporations during the late 1990s. For instance, profits as a percentage of revenues for the pharmaceutical industry ranked the highest among U.S. industrial groups.[12] Nationally, for-profit chains came to control about 15 percent of all hospitals, but in some states, such as California, Florida, Tennessee, and Texas, the chains operate between a third and half of all hospitals. Ownership of nursing homes by corporate chains has increased by more than 30 percent. For-profit corporations have enrolled about 70 percent of all HMO subscribers throughout the country.

While proponents perceive several economic advantages of corporate involvement in health care, substantiation of such claims is limited. For example, it is argued that tough-minded managerial techniques increase efficiency, enhance quality, and decrease costs, although several studies have shown that for-profit health care organizations perform worse or no better on these criteria than nonprofit ones.[13] Similarly, research on corporate management has not supported the claim that corporate takeover can alleviate the financial problems of hospitals serving indigent clients.[14]

Corporate involvement in health care also has raised ethical questions. For instance, there is concern that corporate strategies lead to reduced services for the poor. While some corporations have established endowments for indigent care, the ability of such funds to assure long-term access is doubtful, especially when cutbacks occur in public-sector support. Other ethical concerns have focused on physicians' conflicting loyalties to patients versus corporations, the implications of physicians' referrals of patients for services to corporations in which the physicians hold financial interests, and the unwillingness of for-profit hospitals to provide unprofitable but needed services. Such observations lead to doubts about the wisdom of policies that encourage corporate penetration of health care.

*Public-sector programs.* Policies enacted since 1980 have greatly reduced public-sector health programs. Cutbacks have occurred in the national Medicaid program; Medicare; block grants for maternal and child health, migrant health services, community health centers, and birth control services; health planning; educational assistance for medical students and residents (affecting especially minority recruitment); the National Health Service Corps; the Indian Health Service; and the

National Institute of Occupational Safety and Health. Many federally sponsored research programs also have been cut.

During this same time period, some measures of health and well-being in the United States either stopped improving or actually became worse. For example, a marked slowing in the rate of decline in infant mortality coincided with cutbacks in federal prenatal and perinatal programs; in several low-income urban areas, infant mortality increased. Among African Americans, postneonatal and maternal mortality rates stopped falling after decades of steady decline, many African-American women have not been able to receive adequate prenatal care, and overall mortality rates for African Americans, especially men, remain much worse than those for whites.[15] These reversals in health status and health services, emerging as direct manifestations of changes in federal policies, have been unique among economically developed countries.

Alongside these programmatic cutbacks, bureaucratization and regulation in the health care system have grown rapidly. A distinction between the rhetoric of reduced government versus the reality of greater government intervention, for instance, was clear in the Medicare diagnosis-related group (DRG) program. Intended as a cost-control device, DRGs introduced unprecedented complexity and bureaucratic regulation. By providing reimbursement to hospitals at a fixed rate for specific diagnoses, DRGs encouraged hospitals to limit the length of stay, as well as services provided during hospitalization. Hospitals responded to DRG regulations with an expansion of their own bureaucratic staffs and data-processing operations, more intensive utilization review, and a tendency to discharge patients with unstable conditions when DRG payments were exhausted. Private hospitals admitting a small proportion of indigent patients profited under DRGs; public and university hospitals that served a higher percentage of indigent and multiproblem patients faced an unfavorable case mix within specific DRGs and thus fared poorly. The extensive utilization review that DRGs encouraged focused on cost cutting, rather than assuring quality of care. Moreover, DRGs' contribution to cost control remained unclear, in comparison to other factors such as reduced inflation in the economy as a whole.

## WHERE FROM HERE?

With increasing discontent among the general public and practitioners, health policy debates take on a certain urgency. While an ethical perspective tells us that basic health care for all is an individual right and a societal obligation, the burgeoning costs of the U.S. system hamper domestic economic growth and stability. Meanwhile, millions of people face major access barriers.

Change in health policies to address these problems doubtless will occur, but the specifics of change remain difficult to predict in the complex political terrain of the United States. The last part of this book returns to these themes and advocates local and national actions to correct the difficult problems of access and costs. There is no justification for the continuing and needless suffering experienced by human beings like those whose stories I summarized earlier in this chapter. In this rich and powerful country, we deserve better.

## chapter two

# Local Problems and Global Policies

A THORN IN THE SIDE of those who try to deal with health policy, especially the contradiction of high costs coupled with severe access barriers, involves the gap between truth and power. In a rational world, knowledge about society's problems would contribute to policies designed to solve those problems. Alas, such simplicity in the application of knowledge to policy proves elusive. This frustrating characteristic of policy work crops up in the field of health policy no less than in other fields. Yet the gap between truth and power seldom receives much attention in health policy analysis.

In this chapter, I first describe some tensions in applying knowledge about health policy problems, such as access and costs, to the solution of those problems. After describing the gap between knowledge and power in general terms, I show how this gap manifests itself in two areas of work that hold great importance for health policy on both the national and local levels: community-oriented primary care and small area analysis.

## TRUTH'S SEARCH FOR POWER IN HEALTH POLICY

Optimistically we hope that research might contribute helpfully to the design of appropriate policies in health care and other human services. Almost always, however, there is a tension between the optimistic assumption that rational analysis can lead to rational solutions for social problems versus the realistic observation that the people who analyze these problems usually lack power to implement new policies.

Bearing "truth," for instance, a researcher may search for power and for ways to influence policy makers through research findings about current problems. Yet the relationship between researchers and policy makers, between truth and power, stays fraught with unpredictability and other dangers. Throughout diverse periods of history, researchers studying problems pertinent to social policy have assumed that knowledge somehow would lead to rational policies intended to solve or at least ameliorate those problems.[1] This rationalist assumption pervades the history of research on social problems, and also the history of health services research. Within the latter field, very few investigators have looked self-critically at the degree to which the findings of health services research have influenced policy decisions. In the rare instances when health services researchers have evaluated the effects of their findings on policy, the evaluation has revealed very limited impact.[2]

The gap between truth and power reflects not only the political relations between researchers and politicians, but also a more basic difficulty in logic: that is, the logical relation between positive "is" statements and normative "should" statements also remains ambiguous.[3] Science attempts to validate hypothetical statements by showing that these statements correspond to empirical observations. The statements that science validates are generally of the form "*If* A, *then* B." Here are some examples pertinent to health services research: If prenatal services are provided to pregnant women, then the rates of low-birth-weight infants and infant mortality, and costs of caring for premature babies, decrease. Or, if widespread measles immunization is provided to children, then the rate of measles and its complications decreases. Another format of positive statements involves a simple description of rates or proportions. For instance, this type of positive statement would include the following: More than 70 percent of low-income pregnant women in community A do not receive recommended prenatal services. Or, between 10 and 20 percent of low-income minority children in community B do not receive recommended measles immunizations. Such positive statements describe "what is." On the basis of data, positive statements describe empirical reality and make predictions about what consequences follow from a given course of action.

Normative statements involve "what ought to be." In recognition of the above positive statements about prenatal services or measles immunization, the following normative statements may seem reasonable: Legislators or county supervisors or similar policy makers should allocate more money to increase access to prenatal services and measles immunizations. Logically, however, the derivation of such a normative conclusion demands other normative assumptions, which may or may not apply. For instance, policy makers may also assume that they should allocate money to health services that will improve local morbidity and mortality patterns. But, especially in this day and age, the same policy makers must confront other conflicting normative assumptions: We should not raise taxes. Or, we should build more jails and freeways. Or, despite the end of the cold war, we should build more Stealth bombers to support profits for companies and jobs for workers at home.

True, researchers can organize themselves and lobby their elected representatives to emphasize some normative positions more than others, and I would be the last to discourage them from doing so. But such efforts also must recognize that normative arguments logically derive from moral commitments. In a society not yet committed to health services as a human right, it is doubtful that policy makers necessarily will take the logical leap and translate data about "what is," however urgent these data may appear, into responsive policies derived from our conceptions of "what ought to be." Rationalist approaches that assume appropriate policy responses to knowledge may, with false optimism, divert attention from the lack of clear-cut relationship between knowledge and power.

## KNOWLEDGE AND POWER IN
## COMMUNITY-ORIENTED PRIMARY CARE

Without doubt, community-oriented primary care (COPC) constitutes one of the most reasonable approaches that one could imagine to design and implement local health programs. COPC aims to enhance access to services that directly address the needs identified in local communities. By clarifying those needs, COPC seeks to develop and implement efficient interventions that are able to control the costs of providing needed services. COPC has emerged as a method that tries to apply knowledge derived from research to the solution of specific local problems.

As developed initially by Kark and his colleagues in South Africa, modified by Kark in Israel, and elaborated by a variety of COPC advocates in the United States, the basic method consists of four steps:[4] First, a primary care program defines and characterizes the community for which it has assumed responsibility to provide health care. Second, through local research, the program identifies the community's health problems; this phase of the work consists of a "needs assessment." Third, modification of the program occurs in light of problems revealed in the second stage. Fourth, the program monitors the impact of the program's modification, as accomplished in the third stage. In theory, the COPC method can illuminate the health problems that any community-oriented program could then aim to solve. Yet the gap between knowledge generated and power to achieve suitable program modifications has restricted COPC's accomplishments.

This gap between knowledge and power manifests itself throughout the history of COPC, even in the superb work of its founder, Dr. Sidney Kark. Getting back in this way to COPC's source, one may be surprised to learn a seemingly incredible fact: Kark's path-breaking book[5] about his efforts in South Africa, which helped define the field of COPC, does not deal with the single policy that was the strongest determinant of inadequate access and adverse health status in that country—apartheid. In this classic book, Kark does not even mention apartheid, although this policy proved the main impediment to innovations addressing the local problems that Kark's group identified through epidemiologic research. The same policy proved a motivating factor that led to Kark's departure from South Africa.

Thus, Kark's reports about his and his coworkers' courageous efforts, struggling against great odds to establish a viable COPC program at the rural Polela Health Center, convey a strange aura of unreality, since these writings at no point refer to the devastating obstacles that apartheid actually imposed on this work. In describing efforts to identify health problems, modify programs in light of research findings, and evaluate those modifications, Kark conveys a surprising optimism that such sporadic attempts to organize rational programs can lead to lasting and meaningful improvements among "impoverished" populations like those of black South Africa.[6] Kark's writings do not communicate the enormous difficulties that the team faced in battling problems like malnutrition, infectious diseases, and infant mortality, or the much greater accomplishments that would have proven possible in a friendlier policy environment. The writings also create a misleading impression that COPC, even with less heroic protagonists, can lead to effective programmatic interventions under adverse circumstances. Other writers have depicted the devastatingly negative impact of apartheid on health care and health status in South Africa, as well as the improbability of achieving meaningful improvements while apartheid continued to exist.[7]

Ironically, Israel's policies regarding Palestinians also have limited the impact of COPC in Kark's new home, and Kark's writings have markedly deemphasized this crucial barrier also.[8] Although Israel has indeed enacted a national health program that aims to ensure universal access to needed care, Israel's Palestinian population has encountered numerous barriers to preventive and curative services.[9] These barriers go beyond those experienced by ethnic minorities within the Jewish population, which Kark and others describe in detail. Further, efforts to organize health programs targeting the Palestinian population have suffered from interference and intermittent government repression. Again, the startling feature of Kark's reports on COPC in Israel involves a lack of explicit detail about the adverse policy environment in which COPC must operate, at least in many instances. The implication that rational needs-assessment results in rational program modification by a straightforward process proves misleading.

In the United States, despite its rationality, COPC has not emerged as a powerful force in research, policy analysis, or policy implementation on either the local or national level. Although COPC has received warm endorsements from prestigious government, philanthropic, and professional groups,[10] the circle of COPC proponents has not grown very much in the United States during several decades of activity. This paradox led one prominent observer to ask in 1982: "Why hasn't community-oriented primary care (COPC) swept like a tidal wave over the world and why have not all in medicine embraced the concept as an idea whose time has come?"[11]—a question no less pertinent today. Although various answers to this question have appeared in the COPC literature, the response that seems the clearest is simply that no overall policy mandate exists on the national, regional, or local level for implementing programs to resolve the problems that COPC identifies. In other words, those who bear truths revealed by COPC lack power, or even a regular mechanism to gain access to power, so that suitable program modifications can occur.

All steps in the COPC process, but especially the third step (program modifications in light of problems revealed through a needs assessment), require a supportive policy environment in which new or modified programs can in reality address the problems revealed in the second step. Clearly, initiating a primary care program, doing research to identify problems, and evaluating program modifications (steps one, two, and four) do require time and usually some degree of financial support. But the modification and expansion of existing programs to meet a community's identified needs almost always require substantial investment. This investment depends on a policy-making arrangement ensuring a reasonable chance that programs suggested by research will receive political and financial support.

Without such an arrangement, it is likely that COPC's research efforts will produce a patchwork of reform, where some localities succeed in expanding programs through success in fundraising and/or through unusual levels of personal commitment by providers, while other localities produce needs assessments that remain on the shelf or in cylindrical files. The patchwork nature of COPC's accomplishments without a supportive policy environment becomes obvious from the great diversity of successes and failures witnessed during the 1980s and 1990s.[12]

A critical review of COPC applications in the United States shows that even when investigators have used epidemiologic methods to identify important local health problems, the lack of a supportive policy environment has hampered local efforts to address these problems. Clearly, some successful COPC programs have emerged in both rural and urban areas. Descriptions of these "model" programs point to their organization as primary care practice settings, their attempt to identify health problems through some kind of database, their effort to modify programs in response to needs assessment, and their (somewhat spotty) approach to evaluation.[13] Yet from the rural Southwest to urban Bronx, even these models of COPC have suffered from a lack of suitable policy environment. In private, participants in these programs complain regularly about the remaining burden of unmet needs, the difficulties of translating research findings into effective programs, the lack of suitable funding for program development or even for more basic access to services like prenatal care and immunization, the time and energy consumed by raising funds through unpredictable grants to meet identified needs, and so forth. Yet the publications and policy statements favoring COPC again convey an impression of much greater ease and rationality in the policy process than these private experiences suggest.

Although I self-critically describe in chapter 6 some of our own efforts in COPC, people around the country face such generic difficulties. Some COPC sites have attained outstanding track records of grantsmanship and/or support from government and philanthropic agencies to begin new prioritized programs and to see them through to completion. Many others, however, have achieved only partial successes. At any rate, the long-term viability of such efforts remains ambiguous, partly because the targeted populations are usually poor and thus unable to sustain a program's self-sufficiency over an extended period of time.[14]

Further, even if a COPC site does achieve improvements in a limited sphere, should we content ourselves with incremental accomplishments while so much remains to be done? In COPC experiences, some groups have succeeded in implementing a single or a few targeted programs in response to identified needs. But one should ask: Should we also not be seeking a more comprehensive solution, in which a supportive national policy environment facilitates local COPC efforts to meet the full spectrum of local needs? If not, we come away from the COPC experience with incomplete solutions that convey a false sense of rationality and a distorted image of what actually is being accomplished.

In summary, the gap between knowledge about local problems and the power to achieve responsive policies has received scant attention in COPC. While the efforts of COPC leaders deserve praise, optimism about the success of piecemeal approaches to local problems is less warranted than one might suppose. This situation is unlikely to improve without consistent and responsive national policies to support local actions.

## TRUTH'S SEARCH FOR POWER IN SMALL AREA ANALYSIS

A similar set of optimistic assumptions about the impact of rationality lies beneath the influential field of "small area analysis" (SAA), also referred to frequently as the study of "small area variation" in services. SAA aims, at least in part, to clarify and improve the problems of access barriers and high costs of care in the United States by documenting variations in measures of services and access among small geographic areas.

The documentation of local and regional variation in practice patterns presumably will influence at least two levels of change. First, professionals and their organizations that become aware of such variation will realize that practitioners may be doing a substantial portion of their procedures for unjustifiable reasons. If inappropriate practice patterns are confirmed, professionals will initiate some form of self-regulation to bring practitioners' behavior in line with national "guidelines." In developing guidelines, committees of experts evaluate the research evidence that procedures improve or do not improve "outcomes" for specific diseases. The committees then write and publish the sequence of procedures that practitioners should use or avoid in treating patients with those conditions. Such guidelines arguably help control costs by reducing unnecessary procedures, and enhance access by encouraging the use of appropriate procedures in geographic areas where they remain underutilized.

Second, public- and private-funding agencies, armed with knowledge of small area variations and guidelines set for specific procedures by expert panels, will influence practice patterns through manipulations of reimbursement policies. For instance, payments for overused procedures—especially those that do not clearly improve disease outcomes, according to expert guidelines—could be reduced, while those for underused procedures could be increased, based on assessments of local practice patterns. To differing degrees, overviews of SAA and initiatives to establish clinical standards based on outcomes research convey these assumptions, explicitly or implicitly.[15]

Again, the rationalist orientation of SAA assumes a more or less unfettered flow from knowledge to change in policy and practice. Without doubt, researchers who do SAA studies differ in their beliefs about the impact of such work on the major problems of the U.S. health care system. On the other hand, optimism about the impact of rational knowledge clearly is one reason that SAA has become so influential among governmental and philanthropic agencies that concern themselves with the quality and costs of medical care.

Recent examples of SAA illustrate these optimistic assumptions. During the past two decades, surgical procedures have presented themselves as the most remarkable evidence that clinical practices vary substantially among local areas, without rhyme or reason as far as local rates of illness are concerned. Thus, the probability that a woman will lose her uterus differs widely based on the locality where she lives; so, too, the likelihoods vary that a man will lose his prostate, a child will be hospitalized for his or her tonsils, an elderly person will get his or her inborn cerebrovascular system fixed, and so forth.[16] Without evidence that the incidence or prevalence of diseases in these organs differs across local areas, the variability in rates of surgery reflects at least some unnecessary procedures.

How will this knowledge translate into policy? SAA advocates have argued that professional associations, individual practitioners, and policy makers ought to take such knowledge into account in decisions to change practice and reimbursement patterns. Yet the important findings of SAA should not deflect attention from issues that will limit the impact of SAA on health policy and practice patterns.

First, a lack of oversight and regulation of physician practices makes their behavior difficult to change in a desirable direction. Historically, professional organizations have shown limited ability to monitor members' practices and have proven quite reluctant to intervene when individual physicians become "outliers" whose clinical practices deviate from norms of usual and customary procedures.[17] State licensing boards have shown little interest in or capability of monitoring more than the most egregious violations of legal or ethical principles. Managed care organizations recently have tried to reduce variations in practice patterns, especially when local areas show high rates of costly procedures. However, the long-term impact of managed care policies on small area variations in practice patterns remains unclear.

As to the impact of reimbursement policies, physicians have shown great ingenuity in circumventing the initiatives of public or private insurers, partly by expanding procedures in new or slightly different arenas. Based on the major regulatory innovations of the 1980s and 1990s, which have accomplished very little in reversing the upward cost spiral, there is little reason for optimism that physicians will respond on behalf of the greater good when SAA reveals the irrationalities of their behavior; irrational clinical practices so often prove quite rational from the economic perspective of professional income.

Second, inappropriate physician practices account for a small part of this country's cost crisis—in comparison with unnecessary administrative procedures, private insurance overhead, profit making, and the development and promotion of wasteful pharmaceuticals and equipment. As of 1999, health care expenditures in the United States surpassed $1 trillion annually. Of this amount, approximately 25 percent goes for administrative expenses, which include program administration, insurance overhead, nursing home administration, and physicians' overhead. The administrative sector has represented the fastest growing part of health care expenditures nationally. Profits to companies doing business in health care, not including private insurers, mount up to about 20 percent of total expenditures. Overall expenditures on unnecessary procedures ordered or performed by physicians are currently unknown, but even generous estimates put this figure at no more than about 10 percent of total spending on health care.[18]

SAA's emphasis on physician behavior becomes striking in view of alternative targets for cost savings that lie in excessive administration and profit making by corporations. The curious targeting of physician behavior, as opposed to other equally or more costly components of the cost crisis, raises a question about the underlying values that favor SAA in policy-oriented research. Studies of outcomes that lead to changes in physician behavior remain politically safe, because they proceed from a common assumption that health will improve and costs will decline as ineffective care is identified and eliminated. Here, the assumption is that physician behavior will prove more susceptible to self-policing or external regulation than will bureaucratic or financial interests that occupy such entrenched positions in our country's political economy.

## COPC, SAA, AND A NATIONAL HEALTH PROGRAM

The tenuous relation between truth and power will continue to reduce the contribution that COPC and SAA can hope to achieve. Optimistic assumptions about these methods also may mislead others by implying that something done in the realm of knowledge signifies something done in the realm of policy, when actually not much is being accomplished in the latter arena. From a critical appraisal of my own and others' work, it is difficult to accomplish meaningful change at the local level, even when the findings of community-oriented research elucidate important unmet needs. Without coherent local and national policies that support the translation of needs assessments into responsive programs, the impact of COPC and SAA remains limited.

This pessimism about present conditions warrants pointing out some ways that a national health program (NHP) could offer a more supportive policy environment, which could foster rather than hinder efforts in the COPC and SAA fields. Chapter 7 focuses on alternative proposals for an NHP in the United States. For now, it is worth noting certain elements of an NHP that would provide a strong basis for the success of COPC–SAA. An NHP would not constitute a panacea that would in and of itself narrow the gap between such problems as barriers to access and the power to do something about these problems. Nor have countries with NHPs fully addressed the tensions between truth and power outlined here. Further, the feasibility of enacting a comprehensive proposal in the near future—after more than half a century of debate and indecision—remains in doubt. Nevertheless, it is worth emphasizing some features of an NHP that, if enacted, would facilitate work in COPC–SAA.

First, by providing universal access to needed services, an NHP could ensure that problems identified by the methods of COPC–SAA do not remain merely abstract knowledge. Instead, an NHP organized to take into account the findings of COPC–SAA would create mechanisms so that this knowledge could make some difference in the lives of the individuals and families affected. Specifically, the NHP would pay physicians, clinics, and hospitals for services provided to those in need. The methods of payment would vary depending on the proposal. With universal coverage, the question of how to pay for needed services—whose answer is so often missing under our current health care system after research reveals major financial barriers to access—will no longer plague practitioners of COPC–SAA.

Second, an NHP would provide a national structure that encourages local and regional "needs assessment" of variations in access and health status, as well as a mechanism by which the NHP could respond with decisions about programs to meet identified needs. Regional boards would organize and pay for community-based research to identify local health problems. The results of this research would feed into regional policy decisions about capital expenditures for hospitals, clinics, and outreach programs. Through this mechanism of resource allocation, the gap between knowledge about unmet needs and the power to enact suitable programs could become much less problematic.

More importantly, an NHP could set up a system of annual global budgets for hospitals and community clinics that would facilitate research in COPC–SAA and policy changes that respond to research findings. A major motivation for global budgeting, as in Canada, involves its ability to reduce the excessive costs of unnecessary administrative functions like billing and private insurance overhead. However, another important advantage of this budgeting procedure derives from its encouragement of local research and new program development by community clinics and other COPC sites. Thus, the annual budget negotiated between a clinic and the NHP could include funding to carry out research on local needs and to implement new programs to address those needs. COPC sites then would become much stabler in their organization and operation, as they would rely on a more regular budgeting process to support the four phases of COPC activities: primary care practice, research guided by SAA to identify local needs, targeted programs to meet those needs, and program evaluation.

Such elements of an NHP offer the greatest potential for lasting success of both COPC and SAA. Of course, problems remain in all NHPs, and frustrations would continue under an NHP in the United States. For instance, negotiated global budgets might not be able to fund programs to meet all identified needs, and prioritization doubtless would lead to periodic disappointments. Yet these disappointments likely would prove minor compared with those we presently endure as we work in a largely hostile policy environment. Indeed, without a coherent NHP, local and national politics will continue to buffet COPC and SAA, whose inability to bridge the gap between truth and power then will reinforce the patchwork quilt of partial and incomplete solutions that already plagues the United States.

## INFORMATION TO LINK LOCAL PROBLEMS WITH GLOBAL POLICIES

Linking knowledge and power to solve local problems and to guide global policies requires certain kinds of information, in addition to a great deal of political fortitude. Those who practice COPC and SAA throughout the United States continue to need similar kinds of data on such problems as access and costs, but incomplete information hampers these efforts. While consuming much time and money, national and local data-gathering procedures remain inadequate. For instance, despite the planning and execution of national surveys on health and health services, they often remain unusable for community-based efforts to improve access and to control costs. To conclude this chapter, I want to clarify these information needs more explicitly.

Partly because of the uncertainties in the policy debate at the national and state levels, county governments have assumed key roles in policy decisions about health care access. Likewise, the accessibility of services in local areas continues to depend more on the availability of "safety net institutions," such as public hospitals and community health centers, than it does on existing global policies. In counties whose elected leaders continue to support these institutions, access remains less of a problem than in counties whose leaders enact policies that reduce or eliminate support for these institutions. As a result, local policy decisions will continue to create wide variability in access.

In the United States, we need "epidemiologic surveillance" of access barriers and their impacts. Although much is known about such barriers at the national level, local variability in access at the county or subcounty level has been little studied. This gap in research is unfortunate, because major public policies affecting access will continue to be made at the county or municipal level and because differences in local policies are related to local differences in access.

Prior research is weak in clarifying local variations in access. Governmental agencies and private organizations have undertaken a variety of access surveys. These surveys include components of the National Health Interview Survey, coordinated by the National Center of Health Statistics; the National Medical Care Expenditure Survey, sponsored by the Agency for Healthcare Research and Quality; several surveys initiated by the Robert Wood Johnson Foundation, including the Community Tracking Study; and state-level surveys initiated by governmental or philanthropic agencies. All these studies, however, have occurred sporadically rather than at consistent time intervals. Instead of dealing with local variations in the country as a whole, they have focused on specific geographic areas that were chosen because of convenience or interest to the funding agencies.

Local, population-based surveys can prove very helpful in clarifying access barriers. For instance, as noted in chapter 1, primary care health workers have realized that many patients were encountering severe barriers to access for a variety of needed services. In some situations, these barriers were so severe that death or unnecessary complications of illnesses resulted. National surveys of access, however, did not reveal the extent of these problems, because the surveys were not designed to clarify small area variations in access. In this situation, when I worked with a local group to improve access, we carried out a survey designed to detect access barriers at the census tract or zip-code level. We discovered some of the worst access conditions that had yet been found anywhere in the United States. In chapter 6, I describe this work in more detail.

However, several problems limit the usefulness of local surveys. First, the development of standardized and culturally sensitive interview instruments that can be replicated in many different geographic areas has been slow. Surveys used at the national and local levels have differed in the wording and emphasis of questions, so that findings have proven difficult to compare among localities and with the country as a whole.

Second, especially in rural areas, families with low incomes may lack telephones and therefore may not be included in telephone survey samples. In-person interviews, which help deal with households' lack of telephones, are time-consuming and very labor-intensive. Third, since families from minority backgrounds may not speak English, surveys should be administered in different languages, and translation procedures require additional time and trained personnel. Because of these and other issues, successful local surveys tend to be quite expensive. Given these challenges, it would be very helpful if ongoing national health surveys, such as the National Health Interview Survey, were designed to assess small area variations in access barriers throughout the United States, but the federal government has not prioritized this strategy.

An alternative approach involves local research using large databases such as hospital admission or discharge data. For instance, in studies of access to services, I have collaborated with coworkers in focusing on "preventable adverse sentinel events" that can be used to assess specific access barriers or the impact of local policy decisions. These events can be studied through data that are gathered routinely by health institutions and governmental public health agencies, whose databases can be obtained in the public sphere.

Examples of helpful research using large databases include studies of hospital admissions, incidence of preventable infections and adverse birth outcomes, and county-level variations in life expectancy.[19] Some researchers have uncovered major access problems by studying hospital admissions for conditions that are sensitive to outpatient care, such as complications of diabetes mellitus and hypertension. Through this work, for example, it is clear that people in specific low-income neighborhoods of New York City are admitted to hospitals for these conditions much more frequently than in other neighborhoods. Complementary research has used public health databases to track local variations in infections such as measles that are preventable by immunization, or adverse and costly outcomes of pregnancy and delivery that may be preventable by adequate prenatal care. In addition, county-level data on mortality and life expectancy reveal enormous variations throughout the United States. While some counties rank among the best indicators in the world, others manifest mortality rates and life expectancies resembling those of underdeveloped countries. In general, the counties with the worst indicators are those with the highest levels of poverty, income inequality, and lack of health care personnel.

Again, the limitations of research using large databases derive partly from the lack of national policies to standardize and facilitate the use of this information. Although hospital admissions data compatible with investigation of outpatient care-sensitive inpatient admissions are available in some areas of the country, they are not readily obtainable in other areas. Likewise, the data collected by local and state health departments on immunization-preventable infections and on adverse perinatal outcomes differ in content and availability to researchers. In addition, federal data gathering on health issues usually has included race as a variable but not social class. Therefore, the feasibility of research linking health care and health outcomes to poverty, income inequality, and other social class conditions has been reduced in comparison with that in other economically developed countries. Due to the lack of suitable national norms guiding collection of data and the use of databases, research on access barriers and their impacts remains difficult and sporadic.

Finally, surveys and research using large databases do not capture the experience of access barriers and the impact of policies on communities and organizations. Throughout the United States, safety net institutions such as community health centers and public hospitals historically have tried to provide services to people who experience barriers to access. Although they have achieved major successes in some instances, the capabilities and even the presence or absence of such institutions depend on local policy decisions in communities. While the governments of some cities and counties provide generous support for clinics and public hospitals, other localities provide minimal or no support. Likewise, when public policies such as welfare or Medicaid reform occur, the experience of communities and safety net institutions varies widely in responding to those changes. Although certain studies such as the Community Tracking Study have included practitioners in their sample surveys, these self-reports remain limited.

Such processes that occur in communities and safety net institutions concerning health care access, which are difficult to clarify using surveys and large databases, become much clearer through qualitative observations by anthropologically oriented researchers who can conduct field observations and interviews in these settings. From this perspective, field workers can gather information in communities and institutions about access barriers and the impact of policy changes. Optimally, such work is done in depth and over an extended time. On the other hand, several research projects have been able to initiate brief periods of fieldwork in local communities and institutions, with helpful findings on access barriers and policy initiatives.[20] Again, the lack of a coherent national policy favoring local research makes such efforts difficult and sporadic.

From my own work on local variations in access barriers and their impacts, I have become convinced that a multimethod approach to data gathering is essential. National policies should facilitate research on small area differences. For instance, the National Health Interview Survey, which conducts periodic local surveys including in-person interviews and physical examinations, should be redesigned so that its sample construction and interview protocols would permit meaningful investigations of local variations. Standards for hospital and public health databases also should be determined nationally so that these resources could permit inexpensive research concerning preventable sentinel events in local geographic areas. Regarding community and institutional processes, the National Health Interview Survey could be extended modestly to include anthropologically oriented fieldwork in the sampled geographic areas where data collection for the survey itself is occurring.

In short, just as knowledge requires a clearer connection to power in policy making, the acquiring of knowledge itself depends on the power to create more helpful policies concerning research. With their important potential to address the problems of access and costs in the United States, the fields of COPC and SAA have suffered from the gap between knowledge and power. A national health program would help bridge this gap. Meanwhile, the needs for information on local variations in access and the effects of these variations on health outcomes will not be met until policy changes occur that facilitate a nationally coordinated approach to data gathering and data availability. A proposal for a multimethod strategy to meet these information needs will remain utopian until policy changes occur that will facilitate the integration of local and national research. Such efforts would be a modest extension of uncoordinated research that the federal government already is conducting. The political road to such policies may be difficult, but why not try?

## chapter three

# The Social Origins of Illness: Medical Care Is Not Enough

NOW, HAVING DESCRIBED THE PROBLEMS of access to medical care in the United States as well as concerns about data regarding access, I want to ask about the importance of access in determining the health of the population. In other words, if access improves, will the population's health also improve?

Despite the importance of access to medical care, I will try to make the point that improving access in itself will leave important problems unsolved. Specifically, adverse health outcomes are linked to structural problems in society, as well as access barriers. The main structural problem that determines adverse outcomes is social class. That is, poverty and income inequality are strong determinants of a population's health. Other structural conditions based in racism, gender, the organization of work, and the distribution of toxic substances in low-income and minority communities also contribute to adverse health outcomes. While policy reforms should aim to improve access, such reforms will have limited impact unless they are coupled with broader structural changes in the society as a whole.

Conditions of society that generate illness and mortality have been largely forgotten and rediscovered with each succeeding generation. Now, when disease-producing features of the workplace and environment threaten the survival of humanity and other life forms, it is not surprising that such problems would receive attention. But there is a long history of research and analysis that has been neglected, despite its relevance to the current situation. In this chapter, I trace some historical roots of work on the social determinants of health and illness. Then I describe critically some of the main recent findings from the field and their implications for social change. Lastly, I present some observations on the relationship between the political–economic system and health outcomes.

## THE SOCIAL ORIGINS OF ILLNESS

Three people—Friedrich Engels, Rudolf Virchow, and Salvador Allende—made major early contributions to understanding of the social origins of illness.[1] Although other writers also have examined this topic, the works of Engels, Virchow, and Allende are important in several respects. Engels and Virchow provided analyses of the impact of social conditions on health that essentially created the perspective of social medicine. Both men were writing about these issues during the tumultuous years of the 1840s; both took decisive—though quite divergent—personal actions, which they saw as leading to the correction of the conditions they described. Allende's key work appeared during a later historical period, the 1930s, and in a different geopolitical context. Whereas Engels and Virchow documented the impact of early capitalism, Allende focused on capitalist imperialism and underdevelopment. Although little known in North America and Western Europe, Allende's studies in social medicine have exerted a great influence on health planning and strategy in Latin America and elsewhere in the Third World.

While Engels, Virchow, and Allende conveyed certain unifying themes, they also diverged in major ways, especially regarding the structures of oppression that cause disease, the social contradictions that inhibit change, and directions of reform. A look backward to these prior works gives a historical perspective to issues that today gain even more urgency. The works of Engels, Virchow, and Allende also have influenced a new generation of researchers and activists in Latin America, who also focus in large part on the social determinants of health and illness. I also will summarize these important directions.

### Friedrich Engels

Engels wrote his first major book, *The Condition of the Working Class in England in 1844*, under circumstances whose ironies now are well known.[2] Between 1842 and 1844, Engels was working in Manchester as a middle-level manager in a textile mill of which his father was co-owner. Engels carried out his managerial duties in a perfunctory manner while immersing himself in English working-class life. The richness of Engels's treatment of working-class existence has attracted much critical attention, both sympathetic and belligerent.[3] Engels's analysis of the social origins of illness, though central to his account of working-class conditions, has received relatively little notice.

In this book, Engels's theoretical position was unambiguous. For working-class people, the roots of illness and early death lay in the organization of economic production and in the social environment.[4] British capitalism, Engels argued, forced working-class people to live and work under circumstances that inevitably caused sickness; this situation was not hidden but was well known to the capitalist class. The contradiction between profit and safety worsened health problems and stood in the way of necessary improvements.

Besides his own personal observations, Engels's work followed and made use of public reports to the Poor Law Commission in Britain. These reports appeared in the early 1840s and culminated in 1842 with the appearance of Chadwick's *Inquiry into the Sanitary Condition of the Labouring Population of Great Britain*. In this report, Chadwick documented the connections among economic deprivation, environmental pollution, disease, and mortality.[5]

Engels analyzed problems similar to those Chadwick discussed. Engels's theoretical perspective, however, focused on the profound impact of class structure itself and the difficulties of change while the effects of social class persisted. Considering the effects of environmental toxins, he claimed that the poorly planned housing in working-class districts did not permit adequate ventilation of toxic substances. Workers' apartments surrounded a central courtyard without direct spatial communication to the street. Carbon-containing gases from combustion and human respiration remained within living quarters. Because disposal systems did not exist for human and animal wastes, these materials decomposed in courtyards, apartments, or the street; severe air and water pollution resulted.

Next Engels discussed infectious diseases caused in large part by poor housing conditions; tuberculosis, an airborne infection, was his major focus. He noted that overcrowding and insufficient ventilation contributed to high mortality from tuberculosis in London and other industrial cities. Typhus, carried by lice, also spread because of bad sanitation and ventilation.

Turning to nutrition, Engels drew connections among social conditions, nutrition, and disease. He emphasized the expense and chronic shortages of food supplies for urban workers. Lack of proper storage facilities at markets led to contamination and spoilage. Problems of malnutrition were especially acute for children. Engels discussed scrofula as a disease related to poor nutrition; this view antedated the discovery of bovine tuberculosis as the major cause of scrofula and pasteurization of milk as a preventive measure. He also described the skeletal deformities of rickets as a nutritional problem, long before the medical finding that dietary deficiency of vitamin D caused rickets.

Engels's analysis of alcoholism was an account of the social forces that fostered excessive drinking. In Engels's view, alcoholism was a response to the miseries of working-class life. Lacking other sources of emotional gratification, workers turned to alcohol. Individual workers could not be held responsible for alcohol abuse. Instead, alcoholism ultimately was the responsibility of the capitalist class:

> Liquor is their [workers'] only source of pleasure. . . . The working man . . . must have something to make work worth his trouble, to make the prospect of the next day endurable. . . . Drunkenness has here ceased to be a vice, for which the vicious can be held responsible. . . . They who have degraded the working man to a mere object have the responsibility to bear.[6]

For Engels, alcoholism was rooted firmly in social structure; the attribution of responsibility to the individual worker was misguided. If the experience of deprived social conditions caused alcoholism, the solution involved basic change in those conditions rather than treatment programs focusing on the individual.

In this context, Engels analyzed structures of oppression within the social organization of medicine. He emphasized the maldistribution of medical personnel. According to Engels, working-class people contended with the "impossibility of employing skilled physicians in cases of illness."[7] Infirmaries that offered charitable services met only a small portion of people's needs for professional attention. Engels criticized the patent remedies containing opiates that apothecaries provided for childhood illnesses. High rates of infant mortality in working-class districts, Engels hypothesized, were explainable partly by lack of medical care and partly by the promotion of inappropriate medications.

Engels next undertook an epidemiologic investigation of mortality rates and social class, using demographic statistics compiled by public health officials. He showed that mortality rates were inversely related to social class, not only for entire cities but also within specific geographic districts of cities. He noted that in Manchester, childhood mortality was much greater among working-class children than among children of the higher classes. In addition, Engels commented on the cumulative effects of class and urbanism on childhood mortality. He cited data that demonstrated higher death rates from epidemics of infectious diseases such as smallpox, measles, scarlet fever, and whooping cough among working-class children. For Engels, such features of urban life as crowding, poor housing, inadequate sanitation, and pollution combined with social class position in the etiology of disease and early mortality.

The social causes of accidents drew Engels's indignation. He linked accidents to the exploitation of workers, lack of suitable child care, and the consequent neglect of children. Because both husband and wife needed to work outside the home in most working-class families, and because no facilities for child care were available when parents were at work, children were subject to such accidents as falls, drowning, or burns. Engels noted that children's deaths from burns were especially frequent during the winter because of unsupervised heating facilities. Industrial accidents were another source of concern, especially the risks that industrial workers faced because of machinery. The most common accidents involved loss of fingers, hands, or arms by contact with unguarded machines. Infection resulting from accidents often led to tetanus.

In other sections of the book, Engels discussed diseases in particular types of industrial work. He provided early accounts of occupational diseases that did not receive intensive study until well into the twentieth century. Many orthopedic disorders, in Engels's view, derived from the physical demands of industrialism. He discussed curvature of the spine, deformities of the lower extremities, flat feet, varicose veins, and leg ulcers as manifestations of work demands that required long periods of time in an upright posture. Engels commented on the health effects of posture, standing, and repetitive movements:

> All these affections are easily explained by the nature of factory work. . . . The operatives . . . must stand the whole time. And one who sits down, say upon a window-ledge or a basket, is fined, and this perpetual upright position, this constant mechanical pressure of the upper portions of the body upon spinal column, hips, and legs, inevitably produces the results mentioned. This standing is not required by the work itself.[8]

The insight that chronic musculoskeletal disorders could result from unchanging posture or small, repetitive motions seems simple enough. Yet this source of illness, which is quite different from a specific accident or exposure to a toxic substance, has entered occupational medicine as a serious topic of concern only within the last two decades.

Engels also singled out the eye disorders suffered by workers in textile and lace manufacturing. This work required constant fine visual concentration, often with poor lighting. Engels discussed such eye diseases as corneal inflammation, myopia, cataracts, and temporary or permanent blindness. After an exposition on ocular abnormalities, Engels returned to the passion of his social structural analysis:

> This is the price at which society purchases for the fine ladies of
> the bourgeoisie the pleasure of wearing lace; a reasonable price
> truly! Only a few thousand blind working-men, some consump-
> tive labourers' daughters, a sickly generation of the vile multi-
> tude bequeathing its debility to its equally "vile" children and
> children's children. . . . Our English bourgeoisie will lay the
> report of the Government Commission aside indifferently, and
> wives and daughters will deck themselves in lace as before.[9]

For Engels, the contradictions of class made themselves felt
most keenly in symbolic paraphernalia such as lace, which the
capitalist class enjoyed at the expense of workers' eyesight.

Engels's discourse on pottery workers' "poisoning" was a
clinical description of intoxication from lead and other heavy
metals. His observations of occupational lead poisoning again
are startling, because this disease has evoked wide concern in
modern industrial hygiene. He noted that workers absorbed
lead largely from the finishing fluid that came into contact with
their hands and clothing. The consequences Engels described
included severe abdominal pain, constipation, and neurologic
complications like epilepsy and partial or complete paralysis.
These signs of lead intoxication occurred not only in workers
themselves, according to Engels, but also in children who lived
near pottery factories. Epidemiologic evidence concerning the
community hazards of industrial lead has gained appreciation
in environmental health mainly since 1970, again without
recognition of Engels's observations.

Engels's discussions of lung disease were detailed and far-
reaching. His presentation of textile workers' pulmonary pathology antedated by many years the medical characterization of
byssinosis, or brown lung:

> In many rooms of the cotton and flax-spinning mills, the air is
> filled with fibrous dust, which produces chest affections, espe-
> cially among workers in the carding and combing-rooms. . . . The
> most common effects of this breathing of dust are bloodspitting,
> hard, noisy breathing, pains in the chest, coughs, sleeplessness,
> in short, all the symptoms of asthma.[10]

Engels offered a parallel description of "grinders' asthma," a
respiratory disease caused by inhalation of metal dust particles

in the manufacture of knife blades and forks. The pathologic effects of cotton and metal dusts on the lung were similar; Engels noted the similarities of symptoms experienced by those two diverse groups of workers.

Engels devoted even more attention to the ravages of pulmonary disorder among coal miners. He reported that unventilated coal dust caused both acute and chronic pulmonary inflammation that frequently progressed to death. Engels observed that "black spittle"—the syndrome now called "coal miners' pneumoconiosis," or black lung—was associated with other gastrointestinal, cardiac, and reproductive complications. By pointing out that this lung disease was preventable, Engels illustrated the contradiction between profit and safety in capitalist industry:

> Every case of this disease ends fatally. . . . In all the coal-mines which are properly ventilated this disease is unknown, while it frequently happens that miners who go from well to ill-ventilated mines are seized by it. The profit-greed of mine owners which prevents the use of ventilators is therefore responsible for the fact that this working-men's disease exists at all.[11]

After more than a century, the same structural contradiction impedes the prevention of black lung.

For Engels, the analysis of the social origins of illness was part of a much larger agenda. *The Condition of the Working Class in England in 1844* resembled other Marxist classics in its scholarship, which the author intended mainly for the purpose of sociopolitical action. Engels quickly focused on other theoretical and practical concerns. Despite later writings on the natural and physical sciences,[12] he never returned to the social origins of illness as a major issue in its own right. Yet in a book that aimed toward a broad description of working-class life, Engels provided a profound analysis of the causal relationships between social structure and physical illness.

Engels interspersed his remarks about disease with many other perceptions of class oppression. His argument implied that the solution to these health problems required basic social change; limited medical interventions would never yield the improvements that were most needed. It is unfortunate that

Engels's early work on medical issues has eluded later students and activists. Nevertheless, his analysis exerted a major influence, both intellectual and political, on one of the founders of social medicine: Rudolf Virchow.

## Rudolf Virchow

Virchow's life spanned 80 years of nineteenth-century history, with more than 2,000 publications, numerous contributions in medical science and anthropology, and activity as an elected member of the German parliament. His best known work is *Cellular Pathology*,[13] which presented the first comprehensive exposition of the cell as the basic unit of pathologic processes. Throughout his career, however, he tried to develop a unified explanation of the physical and social forces that cause disease and human suffering.

After a lengthy critique of the defects of detached science pursued "for its own sake," Virchow concluded: "It certainly does not detract from the dignity of science to come down off its pedestal—and from the people science gains new strength."[14] From this perspective emerged Virchow's frequent assertion that the most successful science drew its problems largely from concrete social concerns. Science and scientific medicine, according to Virchow, should not be detached from sociopolitical reality. On the contrary, he argued, the scientist must seek to link the findings of research to political work suggested by that research.

Hegel was the main source of Virchow's dialectic approach to both biological and social problems. On the biologic level, Virchow perceived natural processes as a series of antitheses, such as the humoral-solidistic or vitalistic-mechanistic dualities, that were resolved by syntheses such as cellular pathology. On the social level, Virchow also viewed historical processes dialectically. For example, in 1847, he anticipated the revolutions of 1848 by claiming that the apparent social tranquility would be "negated through social conflict in order to reach a higher synthesis."[15] Virchow used a similar dialectic analysis in tracing the process of scientific knowledge.[16]

While influenced by Hegel, Virchow rejected Hegelian idealism. He argued for a new "materialism" in medicine that would replace dogma and spiritualism.[17] In his attempts to construct a dialectic materialist approach in biology, Virchow cited with approval Engels's approach in *The Condition of the Working Class in England in 1844* and used some of Engels's data to demonstrate the relationships between poverty and illness.[18] During his early years, Virchow was influenced to perhaps an even greater degree by Arnold Ruge, who with Marx edited *Die Deutsch-Französischen Jahrbücher*. Virchow referred frequently to Ruge's writings and speeches, especially those on the ambiguities of political authority and on the need to discover "natural laws" of human society.[19]

Virchow manifested these orientations—of applied science, dialectics, and materialism—in his analyses of specific illnesses. He emphasized the concrete historical and material circumstances in which disease appeared, the contradictory social forces that impeded prevention, and researchers' role in advocating reform. In the analysis of multifactorial etiology, Virchow claimed that the most important causative factors were material conditions of people's everyday lives. This view implied that an effective health care system could not limit itself to treating the pathophysiologic disturbances of individual patients.

Based on study of a typhus epidemic in Upper Silesia, a cholera epidemic in Berlin, and an outbreak of tuberculosis in Berlin during 1848 and 1849, Virchow developed a theory of epidemics that emphasized the social circumstances permitting spread of illness. He argued that defects of society were a necessary condition for the emergence of epidemics. Virchow classified certain disease entities as "crowd diseases" or "artificial diseases"; these included typhus, scurvy, tuberculosis, leprosy, cholera, relapsing fever, and some mental disorders. According to this analysis, inadequate social conditions increased the population's susceptibility to climate, infectious agents, and other specific causal factors—none of which alone was sufficient to produce an epidemic. For the prevention and eradication of epidemics, social change was as important as medical intervention, if not more so: "The improvement of medicine would eventually prolong human life, but improvement of social conditions could achieve this result even more rapidly and successfully."[20]

The social contradictions that Virchow emphasized most strongly were those of class structure. For example, he noted that morbidity and mortality rates, and especially infant mortality rates, were much higher in working-class districts of cities than in wealthier areas. As documentation he used the statistics that Engels cited, as well as data he gathered for German cities. Describing inadequate housing, nutrition, and clothing, Virchow criticized the apathy of government officials for ignoring these root causes of illness. He expressed his outrage about class conditions most forcefully in his discussion of epidemics like the cholera outbreak in Berlin:

> Is it not clear that our struggle is a social one, that our job is not to write instructions to upset the consumers of melons and salmon, of cakes and ice cream, in short, the comfortable bourgeoisie, but is to create institutions to protect the poor, who have no soft bread, no good meat, no warm clothing, and no bed, and who through their work cannot subsist on rice soup and camomile tea . . .? May the rich remember during the winter, when they sit in front of their hot stoves and give Christmas apples to their little ones, that the shiphands who brought the coal and the apples died from cholera. It is so sad that thousands always must die in misery, so that a few hundred may live well.[21]

Virchow believed the deprivations of working-class life created a susceptibility to disease. When infectious organisms, climatic changes, famine, or other causal factors were present, disease occurred in individuals and spread rapidly through the community.

Virchow's understanding of the social origins of illness was the source of the broad scope that he defined for public health and the medical scientist. He attacked structures of oppression within medicine, particularly the policies of hospitals that required payment by the poor rather than assuming their care as a matter of social responsibility. He envisioned the creation of a "public health service," an integrated system of publicly owned and operated health care facilities, staffed by health workers who were employed by the state. In this system, health care would be defined as a constitutional right of citizenship. Included within this right would be the enjoyment of material conditions of life that contributed to health rather than illness.[22]

The activities of public health workers, to whom Virchow referred as "doctors of the poor" (*Armendärzten*), would involve advocacy as well as direct medical care; in this sense, health workers would become the "natural attorneys of the poor." Even with the best of motivations, he argued, doctors working among the poor faced continuous overwork and their own impotence to change the social conditions that foster illness. For these reasons, it was naive to argue for a public health service without also struggling for more basic social change.

Two other principles were central to Virchow's conception of the public health service: prevention and the state's responsibility to assure material security for citizens. Virchow's stress on prevention again derived mostly from his observation of epidemics, which he believed could be prevented by fairly simple measures. He found a major cause of the several poor potato harvests preceding the epidemics; government officials could have prevented malnutrition by distributing foodstuffs from other parts of the country. Prevention, then, was largely a political problem: "Our politics were those of prophylaxis; our opponents preferred those of palliation."[23] It was foolish to think that health workers could accomplish prevention solely by activities within the medical sphere; material security also was essential. The state's responsibilities, Virchow argued, included providing work for "able-bodied" citizens. Only by guaranteed employment could workers obtain the economic security necessary for good health. Likewise, the physically disabled should enjoy the right of public compensation.[24]

Virchow's vision of the social origins of illness pointed out the wide scope of the medical task. To the extent that illness derived from social conditions, the medical scientist must study those conditions as a part of clinical research, and the health worker must engage in political action. This is the sense of the connections Virchow frequently drew among medicine, social science, and politics: "Medicine is a social science, and politics is nothing more than medicine in larger scale."[25] Virchow's analysis of these issues fell from sight largely because of conservative political forces that shaped the course of scientific medicine during the late nineteenth and early twentieth centuries. His contributions set a standard for current attempts to understand, and to change, the social conditions that generate illness and suffering.

## THE LATIN AMERICAN CONNECTION

Linking health outcomes to social conditions has become a key emphasis in the field of Latin American social medicine. Although social medicine is a widely respected field of research, teaching, and clinical practice in Latin America, its accomplishments remain little known in the English-speaking and -reading world. This gap in knowledge derives partly from the fact that important publications remain untranslated from Spanish into English. In addition, the lack of impact reflects a frequently erroneous assumption in the First World that the intellectual and scientific productivity of the Third World manifests a less rigorous and relevant approach to the important questions of our age.

### Native American Belief Systems

For centuries, many indigenous cultures in Latin America have held belief systems linking social conditions to patterns of illness and death. These beliefs often focused on the disruption of customary social roles and the impact of this instability on the health of the individual and family. Native healers frequently directed their efforts toward the reestablishment or reintegration of social relationships.

In Latin America, several Native American societies manifested such beliefs and practices. The most extensive ethnomedical belief system of this type known to current anthropology was that of the Mayan civilization of Central America and southern Mexico. However, many other Native American societies, including the Aztec and Zapotec groups in Mexico and the Inca groups in South America, also developed systems of diagnosis and treatment linked in part to disturbances in social conditions. Such beliefs persist in various countries of Latin America and manifest themselves in such "folk illnesses" as *susto* (severe fright, often resulting from disruption of family or community relationships); *mal ojo* (evil eye); *nervios* (bodily symptoms deriving from psychosocial disturbances); and other similar disorders.

Although the conquest of native cultures by European invaders was as aggressive in some Latin American countries as in the United States and Canada, a greater integration of native and European influences occurred in several areas of Latin America.[26] This interchange of influences, producing a *mestizo* population and culture, permitted a greater openness to social explanations for processes of disease and death. The history of *mestizo* cultural development provided a favorable background for intellectual and scientific approaches that have emphasized linkages among health, illness, and social conditions.

*European Influences*

Despite this historical context of Native American belief systems, most Latin American accounts of social medicine's history emphasize its European origins. In general, Latin American reports allude to the same history of social medicine published in English-language studies. Some of these historical accounts have appeared in widely distributed Spanish translations.[27]

Such historical accounts usually cite the work of Rudolf Virchow in Germany as an important intellectual source for the development of Latin American social medicine.[28] In North America, as noted earlier in this chapter, Virchow remains best known for his work in cellular pathology.

In the United States, social medicine oriented to the vision of Virchow and his followers became one of many conceptual approaches in competition at the turn of the twentieth century. These competing approaches included allopathic medicine emphasizing unifactorial etiology; homeopathy; chiropracty; midwifery and related practices in women's health care; and various traditions of folk healing. By the early 1900s, these competing orientations had created a wide spectrum of explanatory frameworks for education and clinical practice.

At that time, however, powerful forces within the United States began to exert pressure to legitimate a unifactorial model, rooted in laboratory-based "science," as the only suitable framework for modern medicine. Soon after the publication of the Flexner Report,[29] the American Medical Association and the Rockefeller Foundation coordinated legislative and regulatory efforts to reduce or eliminate the vast majority of medical schools not oriented to the principles of laboratory-based medicine and unifactorial causation that the Flexner Report advocated. With this change, Virchow's vision of social medicine declined rapidly in influence.[30]

The historical processes affecting medical education and practice in Latin America were very different. In addition to North America, adherents to Virchow's vision of social medicine immigrated to Latin America near the turn of the twentieth century. In Chile, Argentina, Mexico, and several other countries, Virchow's followers helped establish major medical schools and initiated courses in social medicine. Often these European immigrants worked in academic departments of pathology. As one of several examples, an influential German pathologist, Max Westenhofer, directed for many years the department of pathology at the medical school of the University of Chile.[31] Westenhofer was to become the teacher of another great pathologist, innovator in social medicine, and future president of Chile: Salvador Allende.

Inspired by Virchow's efforts to link pathology and social conditions, such academic leaders facilitated social medicine as a focus of medical education and research. No analogy to the Flexner Report became influential in the Latin American scene. By the beginning of the 1930s, social medicine had become firmly rooted in several Latin American countries.

### The "Golden Age" of Latin American Social Medicine

Although similar tendencies occurred in several countries, Chile's history, leading to what has been termed the "golden age of social medicine," illustrated several typical and conflicting orientations. On the one hand, Ricardo Cruz-Coke, a prominent academic physiologist, became minister of health during the mid-1930s. In this role, Cruz-Coke wrote a monograph that remains a well-known classic of Chilean social medicine.[32] This book concludes with the legislation on preventive medicine that Cruz-Coke presented to the national legislature in 1938, which, in large part, went into effect.

Cruz-Coke argued that infectious and cardiovascular diseases reduced the productivity of the labor force. From this perspective, preventive and curative health services aimed at reducing these disorders promised to boost the economy. Cruz-

Coke claimed that economic reforms would prove inadequate to enhance the productivity of labor, but that improved health care services would achieve this goal more efficiently.

Salvador Allende's work led in a different direction. Although Allende's political endeavors remain better known than his medical career, his writings and efforts to reform medicine and public health made him one of several important influences on the course of social medicine in Latin America. Acknowledging intellectual debts to Chadwick, Engels, Virchow, and other analysts of the social roots of illness in nineteenth-century Europe, Allende set forth an explanatory model of medical problems in the context of economic underdevelopment. This model emphasized social structural characteristics that were amenable to reform at the level of social policy.

Writing in 1939 as minister of health for a popular front government, Allende presented his analysis of the relationships among social structure, disease, and suffering in his book *La Realidad Médico-Social Chilena*.[33] *La Realidad* conceptualized illness as a disturbance of the individual that was fostered by deprived social conditions. This conception implied that social change was the only potentially effective therapeutic approach to many health problems. After an introduction on the connections between social structure and illness, Allende presented some geographic and demographic "antecedents" necessary to place specific health problems in context. He devoted the next part of the book, with a similar emphasis to that of Engels and Virchow, to the "living conditions of the working classes." The last sections of the book presented an exhaustive review of health care facilities and services and a plan for change.

The introduction of *La Realidad* explored the dilemmas of reformism and argued that incremental reforms within the health care system would remain ineffective unless accompanied by broad structural changes in the society. Allende emphasized capitalist imperialism, particularly the multinational corporations that extracted profit from Chilean natural resources and inexpensive labor. He claimed that to improve the health care system, a popular government must end capitalist exploitation:

For the capitalist enterprise it is of no concern that there is a population of workers who live in deplorable conditions, who risk
being consumed by diseases or who vegetate in obscurity. . . .
[Without] economic advancement . . . it is impossible to accomplish anything serious from the viewpoints of hygiene or medicine . . . because it is impossible to give health and knowledge to
a people who are malnourished, who wear rags, and who work
at a level of unmerciful exploitation.[34]

In his account of working-class life, Allende focused first on
wages, which he viewed as a primary determinant of workers'
material condition. Many of his economic observations anticipated later concerns, including wage differentials for men and
women, the impact of inflation, and the inadequacy of laws
purporting to ensure subsistence-level income. He linked his
exposition on wages directly to the problem of nutrition and
presented comparative data on food availability, earning
power, and economic development. Not only was the production of milk and other needed foodstuffs less efficient than in
more developed countries, but Chilean workers' inferior earning power also made food less accessible. Reviewing the minimum requirement to ensure adequate nutrition, he found that
the majority of Chilean workers could not obtain the elements
of this diet on a regular basis. He argued that high infant mortality, skeletal deformities, tuberculosis, and other infectious
diseases all had roots in bad nutrition; improvements depended on better economic conditions.

Allende then turned to clothing, housing, and sanitation facilities. He found that working people in Chile were inadequately
clothed, largely because wages were low and the greatest proportion of income went for food and housing. The effects of
insufficient clothing, Allende observed, were apparent in rates of
upper respiratory infections, pneumonia, and tuberculosis,
which were higher than in any economically developed country.

In his analysis of housing problems, Allende focused on population density. He noted that Chile had one of the highest rates
of inhabitants per residential structure in the world; overcrowding fostered the spread of infectious diseases and poor hygiene.
Again he cited comparative data that showed a correlation

between population density and overall mortality. In a style reminiscent of both Engels and Virchow, Allende presented a concrete description of housing conditions, including details about insufficient beds, inadequate construction materials, and deficiencies in apartment buildings. He reviewed the provisions for private initiative in construction, found them unsatisfactory, and outlined the need for major public sector investment in new housing. Allende then gave data on drinking water and sewerage systems for all provinces of Chile. He noted that vast areas of the country lacked these rudimentary facilities.

The medical problems that Allende considered were maternal and infant mortality, tuberculosis, venereal diseases, other communicable diseases, emotional disturbances, and occupational illnesses. He observed that maternal- and infant mortality rates generally were much lower in developed than in underdeveloped countries. After reviewing the major causes of death, he concluded that malnutrition and poor sanitation, both rooted in the contradictions of underdevelopment, were major explanations for this excess mortality. In the same section, Allende gave one of the first analyses of illegal abortion. He noted that a large proportion of deaths in gynecologic hospitals, about 30 percent, derived from abortions and their complications. Pointing out the high incidence of abortion complications among working-class women, he attributed this problem to economic deprivations of class structure. Again, after a statistical account of complications, Allende allowed his outrage to surface:

> There are hundreds of working mothers who, because of anxiety about the inadequacy of their wages, induce abortion in order to prevent a new child from shrinking their already insignificant resources. Hundreds of working mothers lose their lives, impelled by the anxieties of economic reality.[35]

Allende designated tuberculosis as a "social disease" because its incidence differed so greatly among social classes. Writing before the antibiotic era, Allende reached a conclusion similar to that of modern epidemiology: that the major decline in tuberculosis followed economic advances rather than therapeutic medical interventions. From statistics of the first three decades of the twentieth century, he noted that tuberculosis had decreased consistently in the economically developed countries of Western Europe and the United States. On the other hand, in economically underdeveloped countries such as Chile, little progress against the disease had occurred. Within the context of underdevelopment, tuberculosis exerted its most severe impact on the working class.

In his discussion of venereal diseases, Allende emphasized socioeconomic problems that favored the spread of syphilis and gonorrhea. For example, he discussed deprivations of working-class life that encouraged prostitution. Citing the prevalence of prostitution in Santiago and other cities, as well as the early recruitment of women from poor families, he argued that social programs to eliminate prostitution must precede significant improvements in venereal diseases.

Regarding other communicable diseases, Allende turned first to typhus, the same disease that had shaped Virchow's views about the relations between illness and social structure. Allende began his analysis with a straightforward statement: "Some [communicable diseases], like typhus, are an index of the state of pauperization of the masses."[36] Like Virchow in Upper Silesia, Allende found a disproportionate incidence of typhus in the working class of Chile. He then showed that bacillary and amebic dysentery and typhoid fever occurred because of inadequate drinking water and sanitation facilities in densely populated residential areas. Similar problems fostered other infections, such as diphtheria, whooping cough, scarlet fever, measles, and trachoma.

Addiction was another problem that troubled Allende deeply. He maintained a concern with addiction throughout his career; one priority of his health policies as president of Chile was a large-scale alcoholism program. In *La Realidad*, Allende analyzed the social and psychological problems that motivated people to use addicting drugs. Allende's analysis of the causes of alcohol intoxication was similar to Engels's:

> We see that one's wages, appreciably less than subsistence, are not enough to supply needed clothing, that one must inhabit inadequate housing . . . [and that] one's food is not sufficient to

produce the minimum of necessary caloric energy. . . . The worker reaches the conclusion that going to the tavern and intoxicating oneself is the apparent solution to all these problems. In the tavern one finds a lighted and heated place, and friends for distraction, making one forget the misery at home. In short, for the Chilean worker . . . alcohol is not a stimulant but an anesthetic.[37]

Rooted in social misery, alcoholism exerted a profound effect on health, an impact that Allende documented for a variety of illnesses, including gastrointestinal diseases, cirrhosis, delirium tremens, sexual dysfunction, birth defects, and tuberculosis. He also traced some of the more subtle societal outcomes of alcoholism; for example, he offered an early analysis of the role of alcohol in deaths from accidents.

In his account of occupational diseases, Allende recognized that the occupational causes of death and disability were among the most important that the country faced. The diseases of work revealed direct links between illness and oppressive social structures. Allende noted, however, that knowledge about occupational diseases remained at a rudimentary level, as he reviewed such problems as industrial accidents and silicosis.[38]

Allende also analyzed monopoly capital and multinational expansion by the pharmaceutical industry. In perhaps the earliest discussion of its type, Allende compared the prices of brand-name drugs with their generic equivalents:

Thus, for example, we find for a drug with important action on infectious diseases, sulfanilamide, these different names and prices: Prontosil $26.95, Gombardol $20.80, Septazina $21.60, Aseptil $18.00, Intersil $13.00, Acetilina $6.65. All these products, which in the eyes of the public appear with different names, correspond, in reality, to the same medication which is sold in a similar container and which contains 20 tablets of 0.50 grams of sulfanilamide.[39]

Beyond the issue of drug names, Allende also anticipated a later theme by criticizing pharmaceutical advertising: "Another problem in relation to the pharmaceutical specialties is . . . the excessive and charlatan propaganda attributing qualities and curative powers which are far from their real ones."[40]

Allende concluded by setting forth the policy positions and plan for political action of the Ministry of Health within the popular front government. In considering reform and its dilemmas, he reviewed the social origins of illness and the social structural remedies that were necessary. Allende refused to discuss specific health problems apart from macrolevel political and economic issues. He introduced his policy proposals with a chapter entitled "Considerations Regarding Human Capital." Analyzing the detrimental economic impact of ill health among workers, he argued that a healthy population was a worthy goal both in its own right and for the sake of national development. The country's productivity suffered because of workers' illness and early death, yet improving the health of workers was impossible without fundamental structural changes in the society. These changes would include "an equitable distribution of the product of labor," state regulation of "production, distribution, and price of articles of food and clothing," a national housing program, and special attention to occupational health problems. The links between medicine and broader social reality were inescapable: "All this means that the solution of the medico-social problems of the country would require precisely the solution of the economic problems that affect the proletarian classes."[41]

He then proposed specific reforms that he viewed as preconditions for an effective health system. These reforms called for profound changes in existing structures of power and finance. First of all, he suggested modifications of wages, which if enacted would have led to a major redistribution of wealth. Regarding nutrition, he developed a plan to improve milk supplies, fishing, and refrigeration, and suggested land-reform provisions to enhance agricultural productivity. Recognizing the need for better housing, Allende proposed a concerted national effort in publicly supported construction as well as rent control in the private sector.

Since the major social origins of illness were low wages, malnutrition, and poor housing, the first responsibility of the public health system, according to Allende, was to improve these conditions. Allende did not emphasize programs of research or treatment for specific diseases; instead, he assumed that the greatest advances toward lowering morbidity and mortality would follow fundamental changes in social structure. This orientation also pervaded his proposed "medicosocial program." In this program, he suggested innovations including the reorganization of the ministry of health, planning activities, control of pharmaceutical production and prices, occupational safety and health policies, measures supporting preventive medicine, and sanitation programs.

Many years later, the insight that the social origins of illness demand social solutions is not particularly surprising. Like Engels and Virchow before him, Allende saw major origins of illness in the structure of society. This vision implied that medical intervention without political activism would remain ineffectual and, in a deep sense, misguided.

### Danger and Productivity in Contemporary Latin American Social Medicine

During the subsequent half century, Latin American social medicine has evolved in many countries. For some people active in this field, their intellectual work has proven very dangerous indeed, in several instances leading to torture, imprisonment, or exile. The main reason for this danger derives from the intellectual point of view that social conditions determine patterns of illness and death. To the extent that improvement of these conditions warrants fundamental social change, the perspective can prove challenging to those groups that currently hold power in society. Several centers and investigators—based in Argentina, Brazil, Chile, Colombia, Cuba, Mexico, and Venezuela—now carry out research and programs in this tradition.[42] (The participants and foci of these groups are summarized in the appendix at the end of this book.)

While these investigators and activists have achieved varying influence on medical practice, public health programs, and medical education in their respective countries, they have built an important network of groups working in the tradition of social medicine. For the most part, their work has not been published in English and is little known outside Latin America. Yet their contributions have much to offer in the United States and other First World countries, where the connections between social conditions and health outcomes have received much less emphasis. Such efforts also deserve more attention because of the courage demonstrated by these individuals and groups to continue their efforts under dangerous working conditions.

A theoretical distinction that Latin American practitioners of social medicine draw between their field and traditional public health concerns the static versus dynamic nature of health versus illness, as well as the impact of the social context. Social medicine conceptualizes "health–illness" as a dialectic process, rather than a dichotomy between two static conditions. Influenced by Engels's earlier and Levins and Lewontin's more recent interpretations of dialectic processes in biology,[43] critical epidemiologists in social medicine have studied disease processes in a contextualized model that considers the changing effects of social conditions over time. From this standpoint, the epidemiologic profile of a society, or of a group within a society, consists of a multilevel analysis of how social conditions such as economic production, reproduction, marginalization, and political participation affect the dynamic process of health–illness. From this theoretical vision, multivariate models in public health—such as logistic regression models with disease as a dichotomized dependent variable, either present or absent—obscure health–illness as a dialectic process.

This dialectic approach to health–illness has led to criticisms about traditional explanations of causality in medicine and public health.[44] At a basic level, social medicine practitioners have criticized monocausal explanations of disease. From a perspective similar to Virchow's, simplistic explanations that a specific agent causes a specific disease do not adequately consider the social conditions that either increase or decrease the likelihood of disease in the presence of a specific agent. However, even multicausal models, such as those that consider the interactions among agent, host, and environment, still define disease in a relatively static fashion. Critiques from the standpoint of social medicine have argued that by dichotomizing the presence or absence of a disease, traditional multicausal models do not adequately consider the dynamic linkages by which social conditions affect health–disease, conceptualized as a dialectic process. These analyses have suggested a more complex approach to causality, in which social and historical conditions receive more explicit emphasis.

## THE WORLDWIDE IMPORTANCE OF THE SOCIAL ORIGINS OF ILLNESS

### Social Determinants of Illness and Health in First World Countries

With the coming of a new millennium, research on the social determinants of illness and health has burgeoned. This helpful work rarely acknowledges its roots in the classic studies of Engels and Virchow, or its similarities with the efforts of Allende and current researchers in Latin America. Nevertheless, the recent investigations on social determinants, conducted in both Europe and North America, have advanced knowledge about the social conditions that underlie morbidity and early death. The findings of these studies again lead to a humility about the impact of improved access to medical services. Instead, the conclusions from this field (a brief summary of which follows) suggest that in addition to improved access, basic change in social conditions will be needed if the goal is to improve the health outcomes of populations.

In the United States, class and race remain the most important determinants of the population's health outcomes. Research continues to accumulate showing that the poor suffer much worse overall mortality than the wealthy. In addition, poverty predicts life expectancy, infant mortality, and outcomes from medical conditions such as cardiovascular disease, cancer, and diabetes mellitus.[45] Although the impact of poverty on health continues as the object of research, the findings have changed very little from those that Engels, Virchow, and Allende described many years ago.

Income inequality has emerged as one of the most important class-based predictors of health outcomes, perhaps as important as poverty itself. For instance, research comparing states, counties, and metropolitan areas throughout the United States has found that geographic units with the highest measures of income inequality manifest the most unfavorable mortality, life expectancy, and outcomes from problems such as cardiovascular disease.[46] Other studies have determined that economically developed countries with higher levels of income inequality manifest worse disease outcomes. Researchers such as Wilkinson have argued that the perception of one's economic position as unfavorable becomes a major psychosocial stressor that mediates the effects of social inequality at the individual level.[47] Epidemiologists such as Diez-Roux, Kennedy, Kawachi, and colleagues have developed more sophisticated methods that attempt to trace the multilevel psychosocial processes by which social conditions such as income inequality exert their effects on individuals' health.[48]

Race also remains a major predictor of adverse outcomes. In the United States as of 1999, average life expectancy at birth was about seven years shorter for African-American men than for white men and about five years shorter for African-American women than for white women. In Harlem, survival until 65 years of age for African-American males has been worse than for males living in Bangladesh, one of the poorest countries in the world.[49] African-American infant mortality is more than twice that for whites. Similarly, outcomes for cardiovascular disease, cancer, and AIDS remain much worse among African Americans.[50] Physicians exert more extensive diagnostic and therapeutic efforts for white patients than for African-American patients with similar medical conditions. These differences in practice patterns appear to derive from racially based bias in evaluating symptoms experienced by white versus African-American patients.[51] Again, racial differences in disease outcomes appear to be mediated by psychosocial processes such as the reaction to the disrespect inherent in racism.[52] As Williams and others have shown, the impact of race and racial discrimination on outcomes is often difficult to separate from the impact of social class.[53]

Gender-based differences in health outcomes also are linked to social conditions, although the associations often interact with class and race. While women continue to show overall mortality advantages compared with men in economically developed countries, age-adjusted outcomes in some conditions become unfavorable for women. For instance, cardiovascular outcomes for older women past the age of menopause are similar to or worse than those for men. Although the reasons for women's deteriorating outcomes with age remain unclear, one possibility supported by evidence from research is that gender bias in diagnostic procedures and treatments may reduce their use when otherwise indicated.[54] Gender clearly interacts with class and race in affecting health outcomes. For instance, in cancers affecting women, such as cancer of the breast and cervix, indicators such as rates of diagnosis; mammography, pap testing, and other screening procedures; and survival rates all are worse for poor than for nonpoor women, and for African-American women than for white women.[55] Under conditions of greater income inequality, gender differences in mortality increase, as men tend to die earlier from deaths related to violence, accidents, and alcohol; a "culture of inequality" also leads to more violence against women.[56]

In particular, epidemiological research has documented the impact of income inequality on health outcomes so clearly that mammoth social policy initiatives designed to redistribute income appear completely warranted. To the extent that they would reduce income inequality, such measures as new tax policies, welfare payments, family allowances, and food subsidies probably would exert very favorable effects on the adverse mortality patterns and health outcomes that many studies have reported. But because income inequality is so firmly rooted in the political structure of the United States and some (but not all) other advanced capitalist countries, such drastic policy changes remain a daunting task.

The improbability of basic change in income inequality has led some researchers, as well as agencies of the U.S. government, to emphasize policies that aim to improve the "social capital" of low-income communities, rather than policies to achieve income redistribution.[57] Social capital in communities involves higher levels of social support, cohesiveness, networking, and friendships. Such characteristics do appear associated with improved health outcomes, although less so than reduced income inequality. Although interventions to increase social capital predictably will not improve outcomes to the same extent as policies to reduce inequality, such interventions have attracted support, since they appear easier to achieve in the political context of the United States. It will be unfortunate if the worthwhile concern with social relationships within communities diverts attention in policy away from the importance of income inequality itself.

Access to health care services remains an important goal in the United States, yet it is very unlikely that improved access alone will lead to substantial improvements in outcomes linked to social class, race, and gender. The evidence for this claim also has become clear from countries with national health programs that provide universal access to health care services. This evidence of important differences in outcomes that persist despite universal access again leads to a conclusion that much more fundamental change in the structure of society is required, in addition to national policies that assure access.

In the United Kingdom, social class differentials in mortality and health outcomes have persisted despite the improvements in access achieved by the British national health service. As an example of research in this area, the Whitehall study of British civil servants assessed mortality, overall health status, and outcomes from cardiovascular and other specific diseases during the 1960s and again during the early 1990s. In this research, the subjects all held jobs in the British civil service but ranged from highly paid administrators to lowly paid clerical and manual workers. For overall mortality and outcomes in nearly all diseases studied, workers from the lower income levels did much worse than workers at the higher income levels. In fact, for most conditions, a gradient appeared that indicated a direct correlation between outcomes and social class, as measured by income and position in the hierarchy of civil service jobs.[58]

Class and race differentials have appeared in Canada, whose national health program has won wide international admiration.[59] Again, studies of overall mortality and outcomes for specific diseases show worse results for lower-income subjects. Further, Canada manifests regional variations, with adverse outcomes in rural, economically undeveloped areas, especially in the northern part of the country. These regional variations also are linked with the proportion of Native American residents in the population. In regions with higher proportions of Native Americans, mortality and disease-specific outcomes are worse than in regions with fewer racial minorities. In short, despite Canada's overall prosperity and a national health program that has improved access for people throughout the country, evidence of social class and racial disparities in health outcomes persists.

The maladies that workers in social medicine have described for more than a century remain in First World countries today. Even in rich nations that have achieved high levels of economic development, wide disparities in mortality and key indicators of health outcomes reflect the social class and racial distribution of the societies. In the United States, national health policies cannot afford to overlook the problems that have remained when similar countries have enacted successful programs to improve access. The persistence of these problems implies that broader changes in society are required for meaningful improvements in health outcomes.

## Political–Economic System, Socioeconomic Development, and Health Outcomes

So far, I have considered poverty and income inequality as key predictors of health outcomes. Are health outcomes also related to countries' political–economic systems? The collapse of state socialist systems in Eastern Europe raises some important questions about the impact of social change on health outcomes. Comparing the achievements of capitalist and socialist systems in both health care and health outcomes is a task of obvious importance. Despite much speculation and rhetoric, there has been remarkably little research that has compared capitalist and socialist systems at similar levels of economic development. The widely perceived problems of socialist countries in Eastern Europe, including the political repression that fostered the collapse of socialism during the late 1980s and early 1990s, raise the question of whether the health outcomes in those countries differed from those of capitalist countries.

Although economic development is a widely studied historical process that exerts profound effects on health outcomes, the effects of differing political–economic systems, specifically socialism versus capitalism, have received much less attention. Whether a country adopts one system or another exerts a profound influence on social policy in general and on development strategies in particular. Despite the importance of this issue, there is very little published research that addresses the relationships between health outcomes and political–economic systems at different levels of economic development. Large cross-national studies, such as those conducted by the World Health Organization, have assessed the relationship of economic development to health outcomes without taking political–economic system into account.[60]

In the mid-1980s, Shirley Cereseto and I did a research project, using data from the World Bank, that focused on measures of the "physical quality of life" (PQL).[61] In this analysis, we compared PQL in capitalist and socialist countries, grouped by level of economic development. The PQL measures included indicators of health, health services, and nutrition (infant-mortality rate, child death rate, life expectancy, population per physician, population per nursing person, and daily per-capita calorie supply); measures of education (adult literacy rate, enrollment in secondary education, and enrollment in higher education); and a composite PQL index. We analyzed data for 123 countries, which comprised 97 percent of the world's population. In the data analysis, we compared countries with capitalist versus socialist political–economic systems, within each level of economic development. We also performed multivariate analyses that assessed the relative impact of economic development versus political–economic system on PQL outcomes (table 3.1).

Our data showed that all PQL measures improved as economic development increased; however, at the same level of economic development, the socialist countries showed more favorable outcomes than the capitalist countries in these measures. In 28 of 30 comparisons between countries at similar levels of economic development, socialist countries showed more favorable PQL outcomes. Differences between capitalist and

**TABLE 3.1**

PHYSICAL QUALITY OF LIFE VARIABLES, ECONOMIC DEVELOPMENT, AND POLITICAL–ECONOMIC SYSTEM: MEAN VALUES

| Variables | Capitalist Countries | Socialist Countries |
|---|---|---|
| *infant-mortality rate (per 1,000)* | | |
| low income | 131 | 71 |
| lower-middle income | 81 | 38 |
| upper-middle income | 42 | 22 |
| *child death rate (per 1,000)* | | |
| low income | 25.7 | 7 |
| lower-middle income | 11 | 2.3 |
| upper-middle income | 4 | 1.1 |
| *life expectancy (years)* | | |
| low income | 48 | 67 |
| lower-middle income | 60 | 68 |
| upper-middle income | 69 | 72 |
| *population per physician* | | |
| low income | 19,100 | 1,920 |
| lower-middle income | 5,832 | 638 |
| upper-middle income | 1,154 | 488 |
| *daily per-capita calorie supply (percentage requirement)* | | |
| low income | 94 | 107 |
| lower-middle income | 106 | 117 |
| upper-middle income | 122 | 137 |
| *adult literacy rate (percentage)* | | |
| low income | 34 | 69 |
| lower-middle income | 63 | 87 |
| upper-middle income | 81 | 97 |
| *secondary education (percent of age group)* | | |
| low income | 15 | 34 |
| lower-middle income | 38 | 74 |
| upper-middle income | 59 | 74 |

*continued*

| Variables | Capitalist Countries | Socialist Countries |
|---|---|---|
| *higher education (percent of age group)* | | |
| low income | 1.7 | 1 |
| lower-middle income | 12.1 | 11.7 |
| upper-middle income | 15.7 | 18.6 |
| *PQL index* | | |
| low income | 35 | 76 |
| lower-middle income | 62 | 83 |
| upper-middle income | 81 | 92 |

*Sources:* See Notes, chapter 3, note 61. Further discussion of the statistical analysis and significance testing appears in the sources.

socialist countries in PQL were greatest at lower levels of economic development and tended to narrow at the higher levels of development.

Within each level of economic development, the socialist countries had infant-mortality and child death rates approximately two to three times lower than the capitalist countries. Similar, though less striking, relationships emerged for life expectancy. Differences were again largest for the low-income and lower-middle-income countries, and narrowed for the upper-middle-income countries.

Countries at higher levels of economic development provided more favorable ratios of medical and nursing personnel for their populations. Socialist countries consistently showed higher proportions of health professionals in the population than capitalist countries at equivalent levels of economic development. These differences were again sharpest at the low-income and lower-middle-income levels. The ratio in upper-middle-income socialist societies was comparable to that in high-income capitalist societies.

Socialist countries also provided a higher daily per-capita calorie supply as a percentage of requirement than did the capitalist countries at a similar level of development. The difference between capitalist and socialist countries averaged 12 to

15 percent. Nutritional supply of all socialist countries exceeded the 100 percent requirement.

With the exception of one tie, all measures of education improved with the level of economic development. Within each level of economic development, socialist countries showed favorable adult literacy rates and numbers enrolled in secondary schools as a percentage of age group. Regarding participation in higher education, the socialist countries at the upper-middle-income level showed a greater degree of participation, although the difference was not large. Low-income and lower-middle-income capitalist countries showed a fraction of a percent greater participation in higher education than the socialist countries.

As a composite and derived measure, the PQL index closely paralleled the other findings, increasing with the level of economic development. In all three comparisons within given levels of development, socialist countries achieved markedly higher PQL indexes.

Our analysis of the World Bank's data supported a conclusion that in the aggregate, the socialist countries achieved more favorable PQL outcomes than capitalist countries at equivalent levels of economic development. Were there problems in the data or the analysis that might contradict this conclusion? Statistical information published by the World Bank represented the most comprehensive and accurate body of data on PQL that was available from Western sources. The primary tabulations were readily available in published form for reanalysis. Data collection and reporting from the socialist countries were likely to be at least as accurate as in the capitalist countries. All the socialist countries maintained statistical bureaus that gathered and published these data as one phase of planning and policy formulation. These efforts periodically led to findings that were not necessarily favorable. For example, infant mortality, crude death rate, and cardiovascular mortality in the Soviet Union worsened during the 1970s. In Cuba, reported mortality rates rose during the early 1960s and later improved rapidly; the temporary increase in mortality reflected improved data gathering, as the Ministry of Public Health expanded its efforts after the Cuban Revolution. Underreporting morbidity and mortality statistics frequently occurred in the low-income and lower-middle-income capitalist countries. However, better reporting would have tended to increase morbidity and mortality rates and would strengthen the finding of more favorable outcomes in the socialist countries.

Historically, there was some evidence that the discrepancies between capitalist and socialist nations reflected varying social policies. All the socialist countries initiated major public health efforts. These initiatives aimed toward improved sanitation, immunization, maternal and child care, nutrition, and housing. In every case, the socialist countries also reorganized their health care systems to create national health services based on the principle of universal entitlement to care. These policies led to greater accessibility of preventive and curative services for previously deprived groups. Expanded educational opportunity also was a major priority of the socialist nations, as publicly subsidized education became more widely available. Literacy campaigns in these countries brought educational benefits to sectors of the population who earlier had not gone to school.

Nevertheless, national health policies, including national health insurance and/or a national health service, were not enacted solely by socialist countries. In fact, all the high-income capitalist countries except the United States enacted such national health policies. While capitalist countries at higher levels of economic development enjoyed the fruits of public health and educational improvements, poorer capitalist countries seldom succeeded in implementing such drastic changes in policy.

Cross-national differences in income inequality and the distribution of wealth may have contributed to the socialist countries' favorable PQL outcomes. The socialist countries manifested a higher proportion of income received by the lowest 20 percent of the population, a lower proportion of income received by the highest 5 percent of the population, and a markedly lower index of inequality. Inequality continued to exist in all the socialist societies, but the range of inequality tended to be much narrower than in the capitalist countries.

In the less-developed countries, the differences in PQL between the capitalist and socialist systems were profound.

There, the options in public health and education that a social-ist political–economic system provided seemed to overcome some of the grueling deprivations of poverty. Our findings indicated that countries with socialist political–economic sys-tems could make great strides toward meeting basic human needs, even without extensive economic resources.

Obviously, these PQL advantages, demonstrated through the World Bank's conservative and relatively reliable data, did not prevent the collapse of several socialist governments. Clearly, other factors, including repressive governmental struc-tures and the attractions of a consumerist ideology, motivated citizens in these countries to seek public policies compatible with capitalist values. Several socialist regimes in Eastern Eur-ope manifested very antidemocratic and authoritarian policies. Despite some apparent advantages for health outcomes, the prior political economic systems in Eastern Europe (compared, for instance, with a more favorable situation in Cuba)[62] should not be used as a model for a just society.

Recent reports from Eastern Europe have documented the dismantling of public-sector national health programs, as well as fundamental changes in social policies concerning education, housing, and nutrition. It is too soon to determine how these social changes will affect the advantages in PQL that were observed in the previously socialist countries, but preliminary analyses of data from the 1990s have revealed a marked deteri-oration in outcomes. For instance, in Russia, life expectancy for men declined from 63.8 years in 1990 to 59.0 years in 1993, and for women from 74.3 years in 1990 to 71.5 years in 1993—one of the most remarkable reported deteriorations in the world's his-tory.[63] Recent epidemiologic research has shown that life ex-pectancy and other indicators of health outcomes probably started to decline during the 1980s, before the collapse of social-ism in the Soviet Union and the "triumph of capitalism," but the most drastic deteriorations have occurred after the collapse. The precise causes of this massive worsening in health outcomes, in association with a change of political–economic system, remain unexplained. Some evidence points to the importance of in-creasing alcoholism and violence as sources of early death.

Replicating the cross-national research done during the 1980s, again controlling for level of economic development, will clarify the extent to which the previous advantages in PQL persisted or, more likely, disappeared with the transition to capitalism.

## SOCIAL ORIGINS, SOCIAL RECONSTRUCTION

The social origins of illness are not mysterious. Yet more than a century and a half after Engels's analysis first appeared, these problems remain with us. Public health generally has adopted the medical model of etiology. In this model, social conditions may increase susceptibility to or exacerbate disease, but they are not primary causes like microbial agents or disturbances of normal physiology. Although investigation has clarified the causes of illness within social structure, political strategy—both within and outside medicine—seldom has addressed the roots of disease in society.

Social pathologies—those that distressed Engels, Virchow, Allende, more recent Latin American analysts, and researchers on the social determinants of health outcomes—continue to create suffering and early death. Inequalities of class, exploitation of workers, and conditions of capitalist production cause disease now as previously. Likewise, the constraints of profit and lack of societal responsibility for individual economic security still inhibit even incremental reforms. The links between social structure and disease become ever more urgent as economic instability, unreliable food supplies, depletion of petroleum, nuclear and toxic chemical wastes, and related problems threaten humanity's very survival. Understanding these roots of illness also reveals the scope of reconstruction that is necessary for meaningful solutions.

# ◆ part two ◆

## CLINICAL CHALLENGES IN PRIMARY CARE

# ◆ chapter four ◆

# The Social Context of Patient–Doctor Relationships in the Era of Managed Care

A LONGSIDE ISSUES OF ACCESS, cost, and the social origins of illness, there are important problems of clinical care that
need to be addressed through reform. As managed care proliferates in the United States and other countries, it has transformed patient–doctor relationships in very fundamental
ways. This transformation has occurred rapidly, with little
preparation for either clinicians or patients. In any assessment
of managed care's impact, the effects on patient–doctor relationships deserve attention. The debate so far has raised many
potential problems, few of which have received serious enough
analysis to exert an impact on health care policy, either within
or outside the managed care industry.

The impact of managed care illustrates a more general principle: changes in the health policy environment set a pattern for
changes experienced in patient–doctor relationships. Important
constraints emerge from the economic structure of the health
policy environment. Such constraints include the financial and
contractual arrangements that physicians and patients make
with managed care organizations (MCOs).

Although problems in patient–doctor relationships antedated the growth of managed care, the characteristics of managed care both exacerbate old problems and create new ones. There is no reason to idealize the patient–doctor relationships of the past, but managed care has led to worrisome changes in these relationships. Also, while the characteristics of MCOs differ, structural features of managed care introduce strains in patient–doctor relationships that cut across different types of MCOs. In this chapter, I focus on the connections between the structural features of managed care and the changes that have occurred in patient–doctor relationships.

## GATEKEEPER VERSUS DOUBLE AGENT

Advocates of managed care often claim that this method of organizing services can and should actually improve the patient–doctor relationship. For instance, since MCOs generally assign patients to a single primary care physician, that person presumably can provide continuity and help improve the coordination of services. The primary care provider can communicate about preventive services and encourage their utilization. Since managed care services are mostly paid in advance through monthly capitation payments, the predictability of copayments required for each outpatient visit may also reduce financial barriers to access for some patients.

Not a single research project, however, has conclusively demonstrated improved patient–doctor communication processes or patient satisfaction in managed care systems. The limited studies comparing communication and satisfaction in the managed care versus fee-for-service sectors have found either no difference or observations disfavoring managed care.[1] The adverse impact of managed care on communication processes and the patient–doctor relationship also has received attention in influential editorials and position papers.[2] Further, the claimed advantages of managed care in the arenas of communication and interpersonal relationships have not been assessed in detail for growing subgroups of enrollees, including minorities, the poor, non-English speakers, the elderly, and the chronically ill.

Meanwhile, managed care refers to primary care practitioners as "gatekeepers." That is, such physicians tend the gate, keeping it closed for expensive procedures or referrals to specialists or emergency visits, and opening it only when it is absolutely necessary for preservation of life or limb. The reason for tending the gate carefully is very clear: that is how physicians and their bosses keep enough of patients' capitation payments to break even or maybe come out a little ahead.

"Double agent," as Marcia Angell and others have pointed out, has probably become a more cogent way to think about physicians' role as gatekeeper under managed care.[3] In essence, while continuing to pose as advocates for patients, physicians in actuality work as double agents for both patients and MCOs. The latter organizations hold interests that structurally are often diametrically opposed to those of patients.

Perhaps "continuing to pose" as patient advocates may not adequately convey the conflict. Recently, a primary care physician spent nearly a day advocating for a single patient, a 58-year-old psychologist with a displaced fracture of her elbow, to various bureaucrats working with Health Net, a major MCO, in order to convince them that she really did need an orthopedic appointment today rather than in three weeks, and also really needed surgery in three days rather than possibly in the indefinite future. Many clinician colleagues are burning out with the energy that such maneuvering takes, with such little apparent benefit for either patients or the physician "gatekeepers." At the very least, doctors find that such activities lead to rationing of services by inconvenience.[4] That is, when obtaining services for patients entails such inconvenience, an incentive arises not to pursue the matter vigorously, thus decreasing the probability that the patient will receive the services, even though needed.

More often, clinicians feel an inherent conflict—either ethical or financial or both—between patients' interests and those of the managed care systems for which the physicians serve as gatekeepers. This is the essence of physicians' work as double agents. Clinicians experience this conflict even when they supposedly benefit financially by keeping the gate closed.

## ILLUSTRATIVE CASE SUMMARIES

These structural constraints also affect patients' experience of medicine in general and managed care in particular. The following encounters illustrate some generic issues that increasingly manifest themselves as managed care proliferates.

*A 58-year-old male engineering professor, insured by his university's new self-insured managed care program, developed severe substernal chest pain at 1 A.M. during a Thanksgiving holiday weekend. The patient called the on-call primary care internist to approve a visit to an emergency room, as he had been instructed to do when he signed up for the plan. The on-call physician had covered more than 30 patients on the inpatient wards, in the intensive care units, and by phone that day for his colleagues. He was sleeping soundly when the patient called. He also was a little hard of hearing and did not wake up until a half hour after the patient called, when the answering service again tried to reach him. By that time, the patient had left for the emergency room because of continuing pain. The physician then called the emergency room to approve the visit. As soon as the patient arrived, his electrocardiogram revealed a large myocardial infarction. If the patient had waited for approval, as he was supposed to do, he would have arrived too late for treatment with streptokinase to help lyse the clot in his coronary artery, which was the standard care for a patient with this type of heart attack.*

*A 25-year-old, Spanish-speaking woman who was a hospital maintenance worker was insured by another MCO that workers for the same university can join for the cheapest rate. She presented to the emergency room during her shift at 3 A.M., on the same night as in the previous case, with a sore throat and a fever of 101 degrees. Because she had not realized that she was supposed to call the on-call physician for permission, the emergency room staff called the same physician and woke him up. Groggy and mad at being awoken solely for this bureaucratic reason, he asked to speak with the patient (fortunately, he could speak Spanish), realized the problem could wait until daytime, and did not approve the emergency room visit. The patient complained that it would be difficult to come during the day because of child-care responsibilities, but she could not persuade the physician to approve the emergency room visit, since he had been instructed not to approve such visits for minor outpatient problems.*

In dealing with these cases, the physician experienced several feelings:

- Guilt that he had not heard or responded quickly to the initial phone call from the patient having a heart attack.
- Anger that the nature of managed care led to a critical delay in this patient's evaluation and treatment.
- Sympathy for the patient whose visit he refused to approve because a later visit would prove inconvenient and because she hadn't understood the rules.
- Annoyance that he had to perform mainly a gatekeeper role in both cases, using essentially none of his clinical skills.
- Irritation that financial considerations underlay all these decisions: that he and his colleagues would receive a bonus at the end of the year if they could hold down emergency room utilization; that the paltry $7 per month that two of his colleagues received to cover all outpatient care for each of these patients would decrease even further if utilization became much higher; and that his own motivation to provide services subtly decreased with such managed care patients, since doing more work was not associated with more income. He also thought of the chief executive officer of the second MCO, who reportedly received a salary of almost $3 million, plus bonuses and stock options, and who seemed to be the main beneficiary of physicians' good work as gatekeepers.
- Frustration that all these emotions deviated enormously from those he had expected to have in medicine, a career he had selected with the assumption that he would mainly have the opportunity to serve those in need and receive an adequate salary for doing so, not linked to patients' ability to pay or insurance coverage.
- Most of all, sadness that his communication with managed care patients was becoming distorted by the structural nature of these payment arrangements, and that the openness and honesty he valued were becoming ever more tenuous.

Although as a primary care practitioner I have experienced the above feelings, many clinicians have had similar experiences under managed care. That is why some clinicians have struggled for suitable policies that would not require such conflictual activities and have expressed discomfort with the growing scope of services expected from primary care practitioners.[5]

The two patients in the above case summaries directly confronted the limitations that managed care imposes on individual discretion. In the first case, the patient—though knowledgeable about the rule that emergency room visits must be preapproved to be paid for by the managed care plan—overrode that constraint through a judgment decision about the urgency of his symptoms. As it later became clear, his sophistication as a scientist and educator contributed to his choice to take action without the gatekeeper's permission—a decision that may have saved his life. The second patient acted from a position of ignorance about the structural constraints of the plan in which she had enrolled and could not present a convincing-enough argument to accomplish her own preferences to be seen sooner rather than later. In neither case did the structural constraints imposed by managed care's gatekeeping principle conform with a close and trusting patient–doctor encounter, in which the patient's preferences could guide the course of care in a predictable way.

## FINANCIAL AND ORGANIZATIONAL ISSUES

Also from the patient's viewpoint, the structure of managed care constrains the very nature of the communicative process. Here, instead of exploring possible options with full participation by patients in decision making, the patient must make a case strong enough to be accepted by the gatekeeping physician. Financial interests, by which up to 80 percent of physicians' annual income may be at risk if they do not adequately restrict services under managed care contracts,[6] reinforce the physician's skeptical appraisal. Under these conditions, especially as patients become more aware of these financial relationships, patients' trust of their physicians may seriously erode.

Further, the communicative process increasingly occurs under constraints of time. The on-call physician, unpaid for time spent on the phone in the middle of the night, is not disposed to lengthy and supportive conversation, especially with a patient who is a stranger. For more routine encounters during daylight hours, additional constraints on communication arise, as the productivity expectations of MCOs create standards that require physicians to see greater numbers of patients per unit of time. From the organizational viewpoint, the fixed capitation received per patient exerts pressure to maximize the number of patients seen by each salaried practitioner in each patient-care session. Since MCOs strive to fill physicians' schedules, patients may have to see practitioners other than their own, including physician substitutes such as nurse practitioners and physician assistants; such organizations frequently employ midlevel practitioners to handle the overflow from physicians' full schedules. Physicians employed by MCOs therefore enjoy little discretion in determining how much time to spend with each patient.

On the other hand, the structural constraints in the patient–doctor relationship did not begin with managed care. Under the prior fee-for-service system, communication between patients and doctors suffered from a variety of problems, some tied to the financial underpinnings of that particular form of practice organization.[7] For instance, encounters between primary care practitioners and patients tended to be hurried, and little time was spent communicating information. Interruptions and dominance gestures by physicians commonly cut off patients' concerns. Further, exploration of issues in the social context of medical encounters, which patients experienced as important components of their lived experience of illness, tended to become marginalized in patient–doctor encounters.

The financial structure of fee-for-service medicine created an incentive to maximize patients seen per unit of time and decrease the time devoted to in-depth exploration of patients' concerns. In contrast to managed care, this productivity constraint usually permitted the practitioners substantial discretion in choosing how much time to spend with a given patient. Patients' dissatisfaction with communication under the fee-for-service system nevertheless continued to rank among their most frequently voiced complaints about U.S. medical practice.[8] In recent years, even before the advent of managed care, many calls for improvements in physicians' communicative practices came to the surface.[9]

It therefore would be an error to view the fee-for-service structure as necessarily more conducive to favorable communication and relationships than managed care. The financial incentives of fee-for-service medicine also have created their own adverse effects. Yet the structure of managed care does little to improve those earlier problems and also introduces a new set of constraints that may prove even more contradictory and discouraging for patient–doctor relationships.

## PREVIOUS BARRIERS TO INFORMATION SHARING

Although organizational and financial conflicts of interest are changing the fabric of patient–doctor communication and relationships, several research projects have documented many barriers to communication between patients and physicians, even before the ascendance of managed care. These barriers have derived from differences in social class, education, gender, ethnicity, cultural background, language, and age. In particular, physicians have tended to perform poorly in responding to patients' desire for information about their medical problems, diagnostic testing, treatments, and other aspects of care.[10]

I collaborated with several colleagues in constructing a random sample of practicing internists in Massachusetts and California and tape-recorded 336 encounters in several clinical settings, including private practice and hospital outpatient departments.[11] Regarding information giving and withholding, we asked the physicians to rate each patient's desire for information and the helpfulness of giving the information; patients completed a self-rating based on the same seven-point scale. According to their responses, patients wanted to know almost everything and thought that the information would be helpful, but physicians underestimated the patients' desire for information and, when compared with the patients' ratings, underrated the clinical usefulness of information giving. In 65 percent of the encounters, physicians underestimated their patients' desire for information; in 6 percent, they overestimated; and in 29 percent, they estimated correctly.

One way that we looked at the transmittal of information was simply the amount of time devoted to the process. We found that physicians spent very little time giving information to their patients—a mean time of 1 minute, 18 seconds, in encounters lasting a mean time of 16.5 minutes. After the recorded encounters, we asked the physicians how much time they thought they devoted to information giving, and then we compared this perception to the actual time that we measured from the tape recordings. On the average, physicians overestimated the time they spent giving information by a factor of nine. Physicians thought that they spent much more time informing their patients than they actually did.

We tried to relate physicians' information giving to other variables that we thought might be important. In this analysis, we looked at the time physicians spent informing patients. We also studied the number of explanations and the level of technicality of the explanations. Considering the clinical process of information transmittal, we thought that a possibly effective type of communication might involve the physician's giving a technical explanation and then translating it into simpler terms. This is what we meant by "multilevel" explanations. "Nondiscrepant" responses were answers at the same level of technicality as patients' questions; we thought that this measure would reflect physicians' tendency to respond at a similar linguistic level, rather than "talking up" or "talking down" to patients. The following paragraphs present some highlights of our multivariate analysis.

First, we assessed the relationships between information transmittal and patients' characteristics. We expected an association between information and patients' gender. Based on feminist critiques of medicine, we thought that physicians might give less information to women patients. The findings were just the reverse. Women received more physician time, more total explanations, and more nondiscrepant responses. This finding may have reflected gender differences in language use, as described in the sociolinguistic literature.[12] Women also tended to ask more questions and generally engage in more verbal behavior within the encounters we studied.

Patients' education and social class (measured by occupation) also were predictors of physicians' tendency to give them information. College-educated patients tended to receive more information than patients who did not go to college. Patients from upper- or upper-middle-class positions received more physician time, more total explanations, more multilevel explanations, and more nondiscrepant responses than did patients from lower-middle-class or lower-class backgrounds. There was no difference between poorly educated, lower-class patients and better educated, upper-class patients in their desire for information. However, physicians misperceived this desire much more commonly for poorly educated or lower-class patients. This observation confirmed what other researchers already had observed: lower-class patients tended to be diffident; that is, they usually asked fewer questions. Partly as a result, physicians tended to misperceive these patients' desire for information and generally believed that they wanted or could use less information.

In addition to gender and social class, various studies have revealed the importance of ethnicity and language as barriers to information giving.[13] Regarding verbal communication, interpreting spoken language poses a challenge in primary care encounters. Lay interpreters who accompany monolingual patients often are family members or friends who lack training in procedures of accurate interpretation. In addition to limited knowledge of medical terminology, lay interpreters may experience cultural inhibition or embarrassment in explaining patients' symptoms or in conveying requests for information. Because of these difficulties, the participation of trained, professional interpreters is highly desirable but frequently is not feasible to obtain in primary care settings.[14]

Such difficulties in communication may have begun to improve somewhat, partly as patients and physicians have gained greater awareness of barriers to information giving. The changing gender and ethnic composition of the profession probably has contributed to these improvements. For instance, female physicians tend to spend more time with patients, both giving information and listening to their patients.[15] In addition, female physicians tend to interrupt less and devote more attention to socioemotional aspects of care.[16] Although not well studied, practitioners who themselves derive from ethnic minorities may prove better able to provide information and other components of communication that patients in their communities desire.

## INFORMATION WITHHOLDING IN MANAGED CARE

Beyond such barriers to communication under prior practice arrangements, a new source of information withholding by physicians now derives from the structure of managed care. This barrier to the sharing of information adds to the other barriers already considered. Physicians participating in managed care rarely if ever explain to patients that physicians' own financial earnings under capitated arrangements improve to the extent that they can limit services such as diagnostic tests, expensive treatments, and specialty consultations. In other words, physicians tend not to reveal the financial conflict of interest inherent in managed care.

Of course, MCOs also do not communicate this conflict of interest explicitly to patients whom they seek to enroll. In fact, an infrequent but important source of contention has involved "gag rules" that some MCOs have required their physician employees to follow. These rules explicitly have prohibited physicians under contract from disclosing a range of diagnostic or treatment options to patients when they differed from those approved by the administrators of the organization.[17] The gag rules that have restricted physicians in managed care from sharing information that they believe is important for patients' health and well-being has imposed a basic conflict with physicians' responsibilities under the Hippocratic oath and other ethical norms, which call for prioritization of the patient's welfare over all other concerns.[18]

While some physicians have found themselves in an ethical bind from the imposition of these gag rules, patients have faced an even more precarious situation. Seen from the patients' viewpoint, contracts that forbid physicians to reveal the full range of treatment options or diagnostic techniques to patients violate patients' rights, particularly the right to informed consent.[19] The legal doctrine of informed consent requires that physicians explain to patients the choices available, the risks and benefits of the proposed treatment, and any alternatives.[20] Because a patient's access to this information is restricted as a result of managed care gag rules, informed consent is not achieved, and subsequently, the patient is put at risk. Most often, patients have been unaware that such a gag rule existed and therefore falsely assumed that they were receiving all relevant information to give informed consent for the procedure chosen. Not recognizing physicians' conflict of interest, patients predictably have assumed that they could trust physicians' advice and recommendations because of their ethical responsibility to act in patients' best interests. In such a scenario, informed consent could not be obtained because the patient is in essence not given all necessary information to make a consensual decision. In addition, the consent is obtained under false pretenses: the patient believes that the physician has given all necessary information because it is the physician's responsibility to do so.

These constraints have led to a strange and ethically difficult situation in which patients remain naive about the financial motivations that underlie many clinical decisions.[21] In some ways, this naiveté has become reminiscent of the ignorance and lack of information that physicians formerly maintained for patients who developed cancer or other fatal illnesses. Physicians in the United States used to assume that revealing a professional inability to cure would prove deleterious to patients' morale, and so patients often remained in the dark, even when they strongly wanted to know.[22] All that has changed in the United States over the last two decades, partly in response to the demands of the consumer movement and parallel struggles for full information within the women's and civil rights movements.[23]

In recognition of the ethical dilemmas that gag rules impose, consumer rights organizations have advocated their abolition. As a response, the federal government has banned explicit gag rules for MCOs participating in the national Medicare and Medicaid programs. In addition, patients' rights laws in many state legislatures have extended this ban to private managed care plans.[24] However, even when formal gag clauses are eliminated from physicians' contracts with MCOs, the financial risk that MCOs frequently impose on physicians to limit their services[25] maintains a more subtle pressure that restricts the communication of diagnostic and therapeutic options. Under these circumstances, although formal gag clauses may appear less frequently in MCOs' contracts with physicians, the financial conditions that encourage less than full communication have persisted.

### INFORMATION CONTROL, LAWSUITS, AND VARIATION IN MCO POLICIES

When physicians work as double agents in managed care, one can expect trouble in a litigious society. Some beneficial results probably will come from this trouble, at least for patients and those physicians who vaguely remember why they went into health care in the first place.

Lawyers who work the malpractice circuit have turned to managed care because of its lucrative potential for big settlements. The reason is precisely the financial conflict of interest imposed by managed care on practitioners. If physicians make mistakes, or if it can be alleged that they have made mistakes, it is easy to argue the case that they erred because a financial conflict of interest caused them to limit care to the injured patient. One successful malpractice case, for instance, sought damages from an MCO whose practitioners refused to approve a gastroenterology consultation for vague abdominal pain in a 36-year-old woman who later died from metastatic colon cancer.[26] Similar malpractice cases have been initiated against other MCOs for limiting needed services due to financial conflicts of interest.

Nowadays, physicians, or the organizations for which they work, may assume that to reveal the true financial structure of managed care to the patients whose care they manage would lead to major problems in patients' morale, and certainly in their acquiescence to professionals' decisions to limit services. Therefore, physicians tend to withhold that critical piece of information also. To maintain the advances of the previous 20 years in patients' rights, there remains an ethical obligation to obtain informed consent through full disclosure to patients about physicians' financial and ethical conflicts of interest within the managed care system. From this perspective, it can be argued that disclosure should be a requirement not only for physicians to their patients, but also for managed care institutions to their patients.

A public interest law firm in Arizona asked me to consult on a monumental lawsuit based on the conflict of interest that causes physicians and MCOs to withhold the financial components of clinical decisions from patients. In recruiting patients and their employers, this particular company, like most, promised comprehensive, easy-to-obtain services but provided no information about the financial structure of managed care. After several malpractice cases based on the ill effects of decisions to limit services, this law firm initiated a class action suit against the managed care firm; a successful outcome could be used as a precedent in suits against other firms.

Some of the physicians working with this firm have responded to the suit with an interesting argument, which creates a sense of déjà vu: If physicians told patients that they or their companies make more money when they limit tests and referrals, patients would lose morale and confidence in the patient–doctor relationship. Paternalism thus has moved from protecting the patient's ignorance about dying to protecting the patient's ignorance about the financial motivations in restricting services to the living and otherwise healthy.

The structural constraints on communication may vary across different types of MCOs. For instance, such variation might pattern the restrictions on time spent in communication and on openness about the financial underpinnings of managed care. From this perspective, not-for-profit MCOs, where physicians work as members of a professional partnership (such as Kaiser-Permanente), might exert less pressure on physicians to shape their communication in certain ways than would for-profit MCOs, where physicians participate as salaried staff (such as FHP, Aetna, or CIGNA); for-profit MCOs contracting with independent physician groups (such as Foundation or Health Net) might represent intermediate positions on this hierarchy of institutionalized control over information sharing.[27]

To my knowledge, however, no research as yet has compared communication, or policies about communication, in different types of MCOs. Predictions that organizations with somewhat different financial structures would pattern communication differently remain almost entirely hypothetical at this point. Further knowledge about such variability may come from research, but more likely from a spate of litigation that will address gag rules and other restrictions on communication in MCOs.

## SOCIAL CONTEXT AND PATIENT–DOCTOR COMMUNICATION

One of my research interests in patient–doctor communication has focused on the question of how patients and physicians deal with social problems in medical encounters.[28] The social context of the medical encounter raises important issues for communication in general, especially in the setting of managed care. The following encounter, which conveys an elderly woman's loss of home, community, and autonomy, illustrates this problem.

*An elderly woman visits her physician for follow-up of her heart disease. During the encounter, she expresses concerns about decreased vision, her ability to continue driving, lack of stamina and strength, weight loss and diet, and financial problems. She discusses her recent move to a new home and her relationships with family and friends. Her physician assures her that her health is improving; he recommends that she continue her current medical regimen and that she see an ophthalmologist.*

*From the questionnaires that the patient and physician completed after their interaction, some pertinent information is available: The patient is an 81-year-old white high-school graduate. She is Protestant, Scottish-American, and widowed, with five living children whose ages range from 45 to 59; she describes her occupation as "homemaker." She recently moved from a home that she occupied for 59 years. The reasons for giving up her home remain unclear, but they seem to involve a com-*

*bination of financial factors and difficulties in maintaining it. Her*
*physician is a 44-year-old white male who is a general internist. The*
*physician has known the patient for about one year and believes that*
*her primary diagnoses are atherosclerotic heart disease and prior con-*
*gestive heart failure. The encounter takes place in a suburban private*
*practice near Boston.*

During silent periods in the physical examination of the
patient's heart and lungs, the patient spontaneously narrates
more details about the loss of possessions and relationships
with previous neighbors, along with satisfaction about certain
conveniences of her new living situation. As the patient (P)
speaks, the physician (D) asks clarifying questions about the
move and gives several pleasant fillers, before he cuts off this
discussion by helping the patient from the examination table:

P: *Yeah . . .* [moving around noises]. *Well, I sold a lot of my stuff.*
D: *Yeah, how did the moving go, as long as* [words unclear]*?*
P: *And y'know take forty-ni—fifty-nine years' accumulation. Boy, and*
   *I've got cartons in my closet it'll take me till doomsday to . . . ouch!*
D: *Gotcha!*
P: *But I've been kept out of mischief by doing it. But I've got a lot to*
   *do, I sold my rugs 'cause they wouldn't fit where I am. I just got a*
   *piece of plain cloth at home.*
D: *Mm . . . hmm.*
P: *Sometimes I think I'm foolish at eighty-one. I don't know how long*
   *I'll live. Isn't much point in putting money into stuff, and then,*
   *why not enjoy a little bit of life?*
D: *Mm . . . hmm* [words unclear].
P: *And I've got to have draperies made.*
D: *Now, then, you're . . .* [words unclear].
P: *But that'll come. I'm not worrying. I got an awfully cute place. It's*
   *very, very comfortable. All electric kitchen. It's got a better bath-*
   *room than I ever had in my life.*
D: *Great. . . . Met any of your neighbors there yet?*
P: *Oh, I met two or three.*
D: *Mm . . . hmm.*
P: *And my, . . . some of my neighbors from Belmont here, there's Mrs.*
   *F—— and her two sisters are up to see me, spent the afternoon with*
   *me day before yesterday. And all my neighbors, um, holler down the*
   *hall . . .* [words unclear] *years ago. They're comin', so they say.*

> *So, I'm hopin' they will. I hated to move, 'cause I loved, um, I liked my neighbors very much.*
>
> D: *Now, we'll let you down. You watch your step.*
> P: *You're not gonna let me, uh, unrobed, disrobed today?*
> D: *Don't have to, I think.*
> P: *Well!*
> D: *Your heart sounds good.*
> P: *It does?*
> D: *Yep.*

After the physician mentions briefly that the patient's heart "sounds good," he and the patient go on to other topics. The physician's cutoff and a return to technical assessment of cardiac function (he previously has treated her congestive heart failure) have the effect of marginalizing a contextual problem that involves loss of home and community.

From the patient's perspective, the move holds several meanings. First, in the realm of inanimate objects, her new living situation, an apartment (she mentions a hallway), contains several physical features that she views as more convenient, or at least "cute." On the other hand, she apparently has sold many of her possessions, which carry the memories of 59 years in the same house. Further, she feels the need to decorate her new home but doubts the wisdom of investing financial resources in such items as rugs and draperies at her advanced age.

Aside from physical objects, the patient confronts a loss of community. In response to the physician's question about meeting new neighbors, the patient says that she has met "two or three." Yet she "hated to move" because of the affection she held for her prior neighbors. Describing her attachment, she first mentions that she "loved" them and then modulates her feelings by saying that she "liked" them "very much." Whatever pain this loss has created, the full impact remains unexplored, as the physician cuts off the line of discussion by terminating the physical exam and returning to a technical comment about her heart.

Throughout these passages, the physician supportively listens. He offers no specific suggestions to help the patient in these arenas, nor does he guide the dialogue toward deeper exploration of her feelings. Despite his supportive demeanor, the physician here functions within the traditional constraints of the medical role. When tension mounts with the patient's mourning a much-loved community, the physician returns to the realm of medical technique.

Even before managed care made its inroads into clinical practice, many practitioners felt reluctant to get involved in helping improve the contextual problems their patients faced— no matter how important such problems may be. Physicians may rationalize: There is not time. Or, intervening in social problems goes beyond the medical role. The answers have never been simple, but the productivity expectations and financial structure of managed care discourage efforts to deal with such problems even further. In chapter 9, I discuss in more depth what we should expect from physicians when patients bring up contextual problems, and offer some criteria to guide practitioners in addressing contextual concerns.

## FUTURE STRUGGLES

This chapter has spelled out some of the troubling contradictions that managed care has created in day-to-day patient–doctor encounters and relationships. Under the constraints of managed care, practitioners' role as double agents and the financial structures that constrain open communication have thoroughly changed the nature of patient–doctor interactions. Managed care has created enduring legal and ethical dilemmas in interpersonal relationships that warrant attention in health policy.

Toward this end, the chapter has touched on the unresolved question of what kind of patient–doctor encounter we should be striving to create, as well as some of the struggles that have and will continue to emerge as managed care continues to flower. In these struggles, the very future of the patient–doctor relationship as we have known it is at stake. The era that preceded managed care obviously was not free of problems in this relationship, but the conflicts of interest and mixed loyalties inherent in managed care arrangements have further clouded patients' and health professionals' relationships with one another. A loss of trust and open communication, linked to the structure of managed care, has generated conflict and policy debate. Without such conflict and debate, medicine will have lost some of its most basic qualities of interpersonal caring and compassion.

If the managed care environment has constrained communication between patients and doctors and limited the doctors' ability to respond to patients' contextual problems, the constraints become even greater when patients present severe emotional problems. As many new groups of immigrants have entered the United States, they have tended to seek help from primary care practitioners, often for problems that derive from trauma in their countries of origin, during the process of migration, or after their arrival in their new country of residence. Likewise, due to the widespread prevalence of severe trauma in the United States, many nonimmigrant patients consult their physicians for physical complaints with roots in traumatic events. These issues, and how they relate to the environment in which primary care practitioners currently work, are the focus of the next chapter.

## ◆ chapter five ◆

# Trauma, Mental Health, and Physical Symptoms

MENTAL HEALTH PROBLEMS enter into many primary care encounters—25 to 60 percent, by most estimates—and about half of all patients with mental health disorders initially present to primary care practitioners. Common problems include depression; spousal, child, and senior abuse; situational reactions to such events as job loss, homelessness, and financial stress; severe psychosocial trauma associated with violence and migration; and psychosis (especially among homeless people). National data illustrate the vast scope of these mental health problems in primary care.[1]

Many initiatives have been organized to address these problems.[2] Some of these initiatives appear to medicalize the underlying social problems by treating them as problems at the level of the individual. Few initiatives try to address the root causes of psychological distress that persist at the level of society. That is, the medical model of psychological suffering tends to frame suffering as a process experienced by the individual patient. With a reductionist vision, this model tends to exclude broader interventions that would aim to affect causes such as poverty, job insecurity, financial stressors, urban violence, migration, homelessness, and other social issues that remain beyond what we usually envision as tasks of medical or mental health care.

In this chapter, I focus on the relationships among trauma, mental health, and physical symptoms in patients who present to primary care practitioners. Some of these patients are refugees who have experienced severe trauma in their home countries; others are born and raised in the United States. Such patients often present with "somatoform" symptoms—symptoms for which no organic pathology can be found. Patients with other psychological problems, such as depression and anxiety, also often present first to primary care practitioners rather than mental health practitioners. Yet patients with somatoform symptoms, which can be difficult to distinguish from symptoms actually caused by organic pathology, can present major challenges. Such challenges are becoming an important part of primary care practice throughout the United States, especially as practitioners become more sensitized to the prevalence of mental health problems among their patients.

## TWO CASE SUMMARIES

The following case summaries of patients presenting for primary care illustrate such problems.[3]

> *R.L. is a 27-year-old male from El Salvador. He fled his native country after finding out that his name was on a death squad list for immediate execution. A white handprint with the initials E.M. (for* Escuadrones de la Muerte, *Death Squads) also had appeared on the front door of his house. Nine months after his arrival in the United States, he learned that his wife had been assaulted and abducted by paramilitary forces. His two children witnessed their mother being raped and killed by a group of unidentified men during an attempt to extract information about R.L.'s whereabouts.*
>
> *Shortly thereafter, R.L. presented to a primary care physician at a community clinic, where he was referred from the emergency room of a local hospital. During previous weeks, he had experienced multiple symptoms, including weakness (which caused him to be terminated from his temporary job), changes in sensation, abdominal pain, chest pain, insomnia, and weight loss. R.L.'s primary care physician pursued several possible organic diagnoses by ordering diagnostic studies. He also prescribed analgesics and other medications. After extensive evaluation, no physical cause was found for his somatic symptoms.*
>
> *Psychiatric consultation was then sought. Somatization was diag-*

nosed. Low-dose antidepressant medication was instituted as individual therapy continued. The psychiatrist coordinated follow-up with the primary care internist. R.L. grew more aware of emotional factors exacerbating his symptoms and developed new coping strategies. He joined a group of local Central American refugees, where he was encouraged to write and to recite poetry as a therapeutic tool. During the following months, his somatic symptoms gradually decreased.

X.O., a 19-year-old female from a rural area in Guatemala, migrated to the United States after witnessing the deaths of several family members and friends during military combat in her native country. Since her mother had left for the United States with her two younger children two years earlier, X.O. had been afflicted by intermittent anxiety and physical manifestations, such as tremors, restlessness, palpitations, diaphoresis, and hyperventilation. After she arrived in the United States, her symptoms continued and were further exacerbated when she discovered that her mother's new husband was an alcoholic who initiated domestic violence within the family, and the patient herself was battered several times. X.O.'s native language was Quiché, and even though she was orally proficient in Spanish, she was illiterate. Her limited language skills and education, as well as the fact that her working skills were nontransferable in the North American economy, created additional stress.

   X.O. presented to a primary care resident physician at a community clinic with multiple somatic complaints, including chest pain, abdominal discomfort, pelvic pressure, headaches, numbness of her hands, nightmares, insomnia, and agitation. Her anxiety level had escalated to weekly panic attacks associated with agoraphobia. A thorough medical history, physical, and laboratory evaluation excluded organic causes. In addition, the resident obtained a psychosocial history that revealed her extremely stressful premigration experiences. Posttraumatic stress disorder (PTSD) and somatization were diagnosed as coexisting problems. Psychiatric treatment was obtained; the psychiatrist concluded that her somatoform symptoms were more severe than those typically seen among nonrefugees who experience domestic violence in the United States. The primary care physician and the patient's family cooperated in therapy and as a support system. Initially, she was seen two times a week in individual and family therapy. A tricyclic antidepressant was used on a short-term basis. Her emotional and physical symptoms declined, although terms such as stress, anxiety, and mental health did not seem to exist in her native linguistic repertoire.

These patients and others like them have raised a series of questions. First, how frequently does somatization rooted in trauma occur among people who seek primary care? Second, how is somatization related to cross-cultural differences that contribute to patients' presentation with somatization rather than other mental health symptoms? And third, what are the implications of these issues for primary care practice?

## CROSS-CULTURAL ISSUES IN PRIMARY CARE PRACTICE

Immigrants and refugees, as well as patients from ethnic and racial minorities, present a challenging spectrum of physical and psychological symptoms that is best understood in the context of cultural differences. A cross-cultural approach provides a framework for understanding somatoform symptoms in the primary care context.

First, *language barriers and cultural differences in communication patterns* create obstacles in patient–practitioner interaction that lead to a misunderstanding of somatoform symptoms. Regarding verbal communication, interpreting spoken language poses a challenge in primary care encounters. Lay interpreters who accompany monolingual patients often are family members or friends who lack training in procedures of accurate interpretation. In addition to limited knowledge of medical terminology, lay interpreters may experience cultural inhibition or embarrassment at explaining patients' symptoms or conveying practitioners' requests for information. Because of these difficulties, the participation of trained, professional interpreters is highly desirable but frequently is not feasible to obtain in primary care settings.[4]

*Cultural differences in medical roles and responsibilities* create a second broad barrier to the recognition of somatoform symptoms in primary care encounters. For instance, a "lay referral system" for alternative forms of healing usually constitutes an important part of a culture's approach to illness. Thus, medical practitioners treating Southeast Asian or Latino immigrants may remain unaware of or insensitive to somatizing patients' use of herbal remedies, traditional healers, special foods, or other forms of alternative healing.[5] A lay referral system, imported from the country of origin, may continue to provide alternative therapies in the United States alongside the techniques of scientifically oriented medicine. Even if practitioners become aware of these parallel healing practices, integration of alternative medical roles and responsibilities into the primary care setting may prove quite challenging.

A third cultural barrier in primary care involves *explanatory models of disease*. Medical anthropologists have described cross-cultural differences in explanatory models for physical symptoms and signs.[6] Attempts by professionals practicing modern medicine to explain patients' physical problems may lead to explanations that have little meaning in the context of a patient's culture. In particular, the divergence of scientific and "ethnomedical" explanatory models often creates tension as practitioners fail to take into account patients' understanding of illness as rooted in spiritual forces, supernatural processes, or other culturally shaped events. Cultures also differ markedly in the acceptability of psychological disturbance as a explanation for the experience of distress. As is discussed further below, such cultural differences may help account for somatoform symptoms as a response to extreme stress.

Fourth, *contextual factors* that are culturally patterned may create further barriers to professional–client interaction. These contextual factors comprise social conditions in the family, the workplace, and other institutions, including the religious, educational, and legal systems, that shape patients' and doctors' behavior in the medical encounter.[7] Patients and physicians at times may discuss such contextual conditions explicitly, but most often they appear as marginal features of communication, manifested indirectly if at all. When doctors do not recognize contextual factors, substantial tension and miscommunication can occur. The pertinent social context may include dietary customs, socialization of children, sexual activities, exercise, work habits, rituals, and other cultural traditions that impact on health and illness. Contextual factors, such as culturally prescribed responses to the experience of physical threats to survival during war or civil unrest, may determine the patterning of somatoform symptoms that patients present to primary care practitioners. As an example, for a refugee experiencing the extreme stress of war, inability to protect or to grieve for loved ones who die can create a difficult gap between reality and cultural expectations. When practitioners are unaware of such contextual issues, misunderstandings of patients' somatoform symptoms may result.

A fifth barrier to interaction involves cultural differences in the *emotional impact and stigma of illness*. While many cultures attach stigma to certain diseases, such as cancer or tuberculosis, in other instances emotional disturbance becomes particularly stigmatized. For example, partly because of stigma, Southeast Asian and Latino cultures tend to interpret psychological or psychophysiological symptoms as manifestations of physical disorder and therefore present with somatoform symptoms. Likewise, in some Latino subcultures, emotional disturbances are viewed as both precursors to and consequences of physical disease.[8] Such cultural interpretations of a close relationship between psychic and somatic experiences may prove difficult to comprehend for practitioners grounded in Anglo-American cultural patterns.

Thus, a series of barriers can affect primary care encounters that involve participants from different cultural backgrounds. This model of cultural barriers places into a more general context the specific problem of somatization among patients who experience severe stress, including immigrants and refugees.

## DEFINITIONS OF IMMIGRANTS AND REFUGEES

How do immigrants differ from refugees? Generally, the following operational definitions prove helpful. *Immigrants* are individuals who have migrated from their home country because of perceived economic advantages, professional advancement, desire to join other family members, or other reasons that do not involve extreme threats to safety or survival. *Refugees* are individuals who have migrated from their home country because of severely stressful circumstances, including but not limited to war, torture, forced relocation, or similar changes that constitute extreme threats to safety or survival. These definitions resemble those developed by the United Nations High

Commission on Refugees, the World Health Organization, and the Organization of African Unity.[9]

Federal law in the United States permits substantial discretion to the president and the administrative arm of government in developing operational definitions of refugees as applied to different countries of origin.[10] This administrative discretion in defining refugees who reside in the United States has led to paradoxical situations in which certain nationalities, including Central Americans (like those presented in the case summaries above), are not officially considered refugees, while others, such as Southeast Asians, are defined as such, even though both groups have experienced similar forms of persecution in their home countries. Varying definitions by the federal government, based on current foreign policies, also have led to differences in public assistance, including eligibility for Medicaid and other public programs, for various nationalities. Thus, Southeast Asians generally have been declared eligible for Medicaid if qualified by income criteria, but Central Americans have not. Importantly, the largest group among recent officially defined refugees entering the United States has come from the former Soviet Union, even though not all persons receiving the designation of refugee experienced explicit persecution in that country.

## MIGRATION AND TRAUMA

During the last two decades, sociodemographic changes have created new conditions for health and mental health practices in the United States. Features of both immigrants and refugees may be found among migrating groups. A substantial increase of immigrants and refugees has occurred during recent years in the United States. Table 5.1 illustrates these changes through census data between 1980 and 1990 (the last census available at the time of this writing). Although census data do not differentiate between immigrants and refugees, certain general conclusions can be reached based on country of origin. Regarding the Latino population, the Mexican community grew from 8,678,632 in 1980 to 13,495,938 in 1990—a 56 percent increase. Latinos categorized as "other" increased by 64 percent during the same time interval.[11] This "other" category is represented mainly by

**TABLE 5.1**

MINORITY GROUPS IN THE UNITED STATES, BY NATIONALITY

|  | 1980 | 1990 | % Change |
|---|---|---|---|
| **HISPANICS** | | | |
| Mexican | 8,678,632 | 13,495,938 | 56 |
| Puerto Rican | 2,004,961 | 2,727,754 | 37 |
| Cuban | 806,223 | 1,043,932 | 30 |
| Other | 3,113,867 | 5,086,435 | 64 |
| **ASIANS** | | | |
| Chinese | 812,178 | 1,645,472 | 103 |
| Filipino | 781,894 | 1,406,770 | 77 |
| Japanese | 716,331 | 847,562 | 19 |
| Asian Indian | 387,223 | 815,447 | 111 |
| Korean | 357,393 | 798,849 | 124 |
| Vietnamese | 245,025 | 614,547 | 151 |

*Sources:* See Note 11.

people from El Salvador, Guatemala, Nicaragua, and some other South American and Caribbean countries. Major increases in the Asian population also have occurred.

During the 1980s and 1990s, Central America has been recognized as a region of war where multiple political and economic changes have taken place. El Salvador's civil war, for example, has displaced 10 percent of the entire population within the country, or 500,000 people. Additionally, 750,000 to 1,000,000 Salvadoreans have fled their homeland.[12]

Traumatic experiences in countries of origin may predispose refugees to heightened help-seeking behavior and somatization. Central Americans coming to the United States may face substantial psychosocial trauma. Many of them previously have experienced warfare, political persecution, economic hardship, incarceration, or injury. Central Americans have been at risk of experiencing adjustment difficulties following their arrival in the United States.[13]

For refugees from Southeast Asia and the former Soviet Union with limited prior exposure to Western culture, immersion into new social, political, and economic structures may exacerbate their premigration trauma.[14] This experience may result in psychosocial distress manifested through somatization, which is an important clinical feature in many Southeast Asian refugees' presentation to primary care practitioners.[15] A negative stigma often is attached to mental illness in Asian cultures. Somatic responses then can become more socially acceptable than explicit psychological expressions of emotional distress. Similar observations of heightened help-seeking behavior and somatoform symptoms have occurred among refugees from the former Soviet Union. In particular, Jewish refugees from the Soviet Union have preferred to consult primary care practitioners for mental health services.[16]

Experiences in the country of origin may precede stressful experiences in the country of refuge, such as attempts to find political asylum, refugee camps, new family relations, different language, lack of relevant work skills, and elimination of social-support systems. Such experiences may result in emotional disturbances and also somatoform symptoms that prove to have no organic basis. Anxiety, depression, delayed grief, and PTSD may emerge as specific emotional reactions to refugee trauma. The development of both emotional and somatoform responses to traumatic experiences may be delayed until a refugee reaches the country of resettlement.

Somatization is a common idiom of help-seeking behavior in the general U.S. population. A substantial proportion of patients' visits in primary care, estimated at more than 25 percent, involves somatic complaints linked to underlying psychological distress.[17] Thus, somatization occurs across cultural boundaries and clearly is not a clinical feature exhibited only by the immigrant and refugee population.

Cross-cultural research involving these populations in the primary care setting remains limited. For instance, an influential review categorized the mechanisms of somatization according to currently held neurobiologic, psychodynamic, behavioral, and sociocultural theories;[18] this review did not refer to somatization in refugees, or to the impact of extremely stressful experiences on the development and presentation of somatoform symptoms. A monograph on somatization disorder, commissioned by the National Institute of Mental Health (NIMH), reviewed the history, mechanisms, prevalence, and clinical features of the disorder but did not emphasize cross-cultural differences, acculturation, or PTSD as a possible comorbid disorder or as a disorder to be considered in the differential diagnosis of somatization.[19] The American Psychiatric Association's official diagnostic manual indicated that victims of extraordinary experiences such as natural disasters, accidents, torture, and war-related incidents are predisposed to PTSD, but did not comment on the relationship between somatization and PTSD.[20] Similarly, a major historical review of psychosomatic illness did not mention such an association.[21]

### SOMATOFORM SYMPTOMS, CULTURE, AND PRIMARY CARE UTILIZATION

The diagnosis of the somatoform disorders is not straightforward, in either psychiatric or primary care settings. Because of such ambiguities, the primary care practitioner faces considerable difficulty in reaching an appropriate diagnosis. The *Diagnostic and Statistical Manual of Mental Disorders (DSM-IV)*,[22] the official diagnostic reference of the American Psychiatric Association, contains rather severe limitations. *DSM* has defined six types of somatoform disorders that presume no other primary psychiatric disorder but may manifest clinical features that overlap with anxiety and depression; several changes in definitions occurred between *DSM-IV* and the prior edition, *DSM-III-R*. The *DSM* indicates that somatization is a long-standing pattern of illness behavior, a way of life dominated by medical experiences and possibly disturbed personal relationships.

There is little indication in *DSM* of the possibility that physical symptoms may be at least partly sociosomatic in nature—that is, manifestations of socioeconomic, environmental, or political stress, particularly in relation to war. In addition, PTSD is regarded as a disorder resulting from exposure to a traumatic event that is *outside* the range of normal experience. Such events include combat, torture, natural disasters such as floods or earthquakes, and accidental disasters such as airplane crashes. Contrary to these clinical assumptions, in countries such as El Salvador, Guatemala, Nicaragua, and several Southeast Asian nations, war has become a formal practice *within* the range of normal daily experience, including both combat and torture.

The prevalence of somatization varies across cultures. In an early cross-cultural comparison, Italian Americans complained more often than Irish Americans about somatic symptoms, and their symptoms involved more bodily areas.[23] Studies involving Middle Eastern and Asian patients have noted the importance of culture and the impact of acculturation following the experience of migration on somatoform symptoms.[24] The presentation of somatoform complaints appears to differ among Southeast Asian ethnic groups.[25] Further, somatization shows a relatively high prevalence among Latino respondents in the United States, although the prevalence rates vary among subgroups of the Latino population (Mexican American, Puerto Rican, and Cuban American).[26] Predictably, the degree of acculturation to a new culture after immigration may mediate the relationship between culture and somatization.

Partly because patients with somatization use medical services more frequently than nonsomatizers, management of somatization can prove difficult and expensive.[27] Even though access to care is not always available to minorities, it may be expected that somatization among at-risk cultural groups also would lead to greater health care utilization and costs. Some studies have indicated that per-capita expenditures for hospital services among patients with somatization greatly exceed the average per-capita amount in the United States.[28]

It is often presumed that patients who somatize use services differently and in more costly ways than patients who do not. Relatively little information is available about these problems in primary care settings, however, especially those that attract patients from culturally diverse and minority backgrounds. Such patients are at a higher risk of misdiagnosis as well as inappropriate diagnostic or therapeutic interventions by physicians who are not sensitized to culturally based somatoform symptoms.

## TRAUMA, NARRATIVE, AND SOMATOFORM SYMPTOMS

Perhaps more than in other clinical conditions, recognition and treatment of somatization requires attention to the cross-cultural issues in primary care practice. Language and cultural differences in communication patterns lead to cross-cultural variations in the prevalence of somatoform symptoms, which make their recognition more difficult for primary care practitioners. To the extent that cultures differ in medical roles and responsibilities, patients who have experienced alternative healing practices may encounter disappointments when practitioners trained in Western medical traditions respond with technical studies and treatments for somatoform symptoms with major cultural or psychosocial components. Likewise, when patients hold culturally determined explanatory models of disease, their expectations for medical intervention in somatoform conditions may conflict markedly with those of practitioners who are unaware of cultural differences in explanatory models. Contextual factors, especially traumas such as those provoked by war, civil unrest, and difficulties in migration, also affect the development of somatoform symptoms. In addition, reflecting cultural variation in the emotional impact and stigma of symptoms, several immigrant cultures encourage the interpretation of psychological symptoms as manifestations of somatic disorders.

How is extreme stress processed psychologically, and how is this process mediated by culture? Narrative is a useful conceptual focus in trying to answer this question. As a start, one might postulate that extreme stress (such as torture, rape, witnessing deaths of relatives, forced migration, and sexual abuse) is processed psychologically as a terrible narrative, a narrative of events too awful to hold in conscious memory, a narrative that cannot be told coherently in the internal storytelling of everyday consciousness, a narrative so terrifying that it must somehow be transformed. Within traditional psychoanalysis, "repression" or "displacement" or "dissociation" are psychologic defenses against the terrible narrative, and "hysteria" the predictable result. Yet such terms scarcely appear adequate to describe the psychic processing of overwhelming stress and the appearance of somatoform symptoms in persons who otherwise show little or no evidence of the usual "neurotic" features evoked by these terms.

Another case history illustrates the process of how incomplete narratives provide a linkage between severe trauma and somatoform symptoms. The patient here is a young woman from Native American and Latino cultural traditions. Similar psychosocial processes, however, occur among refugees from other countries and among many nonminority patients in the United States who have suffered severe trauma. The patient agreed to cooperate in a large study of mental health issues in primary care. In this study, subjects who sought primary care services participated in a structured psychiatric interview (the Composite International Diagnostic Interview, CIDI, an instrument developed by the World Health Organization to be used across cultures and languages), as well as a clinical interview conducted by a psychologist.

> A 34-year-old Chicana woman, born in the United States of Latino and Native American descent, came to the clinic for treatment of vaginal itching and discharge and pelvic pain. During the encounter with her physician, she makes no reference to symptoms outside the pelvis. Although the physician does not elicit further somatic symptoms during the first encounter, the CIDI, given by a research assistant, identifies five symptoms in four organ systems that remain unexplained. In the structured instrument, however, little information emerges about the details of the traumatic experiences in her life or about how these experiences might be related to her unexplained somatic complaints.

Not until the in-depth clinical interview, given by a trained psychologist, does the patient's narrative of trauma and somatic symptoms emerge in a clear way, although even here the narrative remains fragmented and incomplete. The incoherence of the narrative combines with explicit references to cultural beliefs, including an "Indian voice" that protects her from emotional and physical harm. The following notes, prepared by the psychologist, summarize pertinent parts of the clinical interview:

> In brief, this patient has experienced a long series of psychosocial traumas, which included sexual and physical abuse during childhood and two marriages. When the patient was six years old, her mother went to

*prison. During the mother's absence, she lived with various relatives and was physically abused in one home and sexually molested in another. She was in a serious car accident at age 16, the same year that she married and had a child. Her husband was physically abusive, and she left him, only to marry another abusive man. She left the second husband when he pulled a gun on her and threatened to kill her. At the time of the interview, she was keeping her whereabouts a secret, as his threats to kill her had continued after the separation.*

*This patient has suffered from multiple illnesses and somatic complaints since early childhood and has undergone ten surgeries. Currently she complains of eight symptoms and suffers from six physical illnesses. In particular, she describes having had severe headaches since childhood. When she was young, they were so bad that they caused her to lose memory and to remain fatigued for several days. She vehemently denies, however, that there is any connection between her health problems and the stresses that she has experienced.*

*Since childhood, the patient has heard voices. When the voices talk to her, sometimes it feels as if she is in a trance. If too many of them are talking, they make her head hurt. She often writes down what the voices say and she has noticed that the handwriting she uses has several distinct styles. Some of the voices are able to spell perfectly, although ordinarily she is a poor speller. She describes an "Indian" voice that protects her and explains this in the context of information that her grandmother has shared with her about good spirits that "don't try to get in your body, but only talk to your mind." The Indian voice has protected her throughout her life.*

*Although the patient draws a link between headaches and the voices (she states that her head hurts when too many of the voices are talking to her), she does not draw a causal link between the headaches and any of the abuses that she has experienced. She describes her symptoms and experiences in a disjointed and dreamlike fashion.*

Later during the interview, the psychologist (interviewer, I) elicits eight symptoms that remain unexplained, including severe headaches. At this point, the patient (P) describes the onset of the headaches during childhood, as well as the technical diagnostic measures that were initiated, leading to the diagnosis of migraine. Although the headaches do manifest some characteristics of classic migraine, which include vomiting, they also are associated with evidence of dissociation, such as memory loss and exhaustion, which split off the painful memories from consciousness. For this patient, the presence of voices, and especially a culturally patterned Indian voice, shapes the interrelationships among trauma, culture, and somatoform symptoms. At a conscious level, the patient does not connect the headaches, voices, and sexual abuse that she was experiencing at that time:

I:  *How was your health in childhood? Did you have any . . .*
P:  *Yeah.*
I:  *You were sick a lot, what kinds of problems?*
P:  *I had hepatitis and* [words unclear] *in '68, I was in the hospital for a month, I had epilepsy attacks, they were giving me medication three times a day but then they stopped because* [words unclear] . . .
I:  [words unclear] . . .
P:  *I was feeling migraines or pressure, 'cause you know I was little I fell off the seesaw and I had like a little pebble, a little piece of rock or a little pebble there, you know,* [words unclear] *so I had those* [words unclear] *where they put the needles, not needles, uh . . . CAT scan,* [words unclear] *all different stuff, because they thought it was a tumor.*
I:  *Okay.*
P:  *And I'd get real bad headaches, I mean super! And they I'd just vomit . . .*
I:  *Is this when you were little?*
P:  *Uh-huh. I'd vomit and I don't remember anything and uh . . . it was like an epilepsy attack.*
I:  *So your headaches caused you to vomit and lose memory?*
P:  *Yes, like tired for three days, now I can control it 'cause I'm older but for three days I'm like exhausted, pressure under the eyes, the cheekbones and then I have a real bad sinus.*

The patient's narrative is fragmented and incomplete. She has experienced numerous stressful and traumatic events throughout her life. These events come to light during different phases of the in-depth interview with a psychologist and receive no mention at all during the encounter with her primary care physician. The traumatic events and the physical symptoms remain unconnected in the patient's and in the physician's consciousness.

Culture does, however, influence the coping mechanisms

that this patient uses, in the form of the "Indian voice" that the patient feels protects her, a voice originating for the patient in Native American beliefs about good and bad spirits. Here, the processing of trauma and culture involves an incomplete or incoherent narrative of childhood experiences and traditional teachings. The culturally influenced narrative does not completely incorporate the extent of this patient's traumatic experiences. Yet the protective voice can be thought of as a culturally influenced narrative that has helped this patient function on a daily basis, even though it may not have been capable of helping her process the trauma sufficiently to alleviate the multiple physical and psychological symptoms that she experiences. This narrative remains an unspoken link to physical symptoms that continue to trouble the patient in ways inaccessible to medical intervention, despite her many attempts to seek solutions in the medical sphere. Eliciting the narrative requires a method that permits in-depth probing, well beyond that of the standard medical or research interview.

Culture patterns the characteristic psychological and somatic processing of the terrible narrative. In some cultures, overt psychological breakdown and the stopping of participation in customary social roles may be a preferred "way of knowing" a narrative too terrible to tell. In other cultures, such psychological symptoms may be discouraged, and maintenance of customary social roles may be encouraged normatively even in the face of overwhelming stress. In the latter cultural context, the terrible narrative then may be transformed into somatic symptoms.

I would argue that the mechanism by which trauma is transformed into somatic symptoms often involves an incoherence in narrative structure, because of which the traumatic experience cannot be told as a coherent whole. This argument recognizes the substantial variability that manifests itself in the connections among trauma, culture, and somatization. Patients who have experienced trauma constitute only a subset of somatizing patients. Further, somatization often may occur as a comorbid condition along with such disorders as depression or anxiety, even though cultural norms may predispose to the appearance of somatic as opposed to psychological symptoms for most members of the culture who experience severe trauma.[29] Yet the narrative structure and its coherence versus incoherence may provide a link among trauma, culture, and somatization in many patients whose physical symptoms cannot be explained by physical disease.

How specific symptoms present themselves also depends partly on how culture patterns their expression. For instance, in Southeast Asian cultures, which place high esteem and positive evaluation on the head, traumatic experiences associated with war and imprisonment predictably would manifest themselves as symptoms of headache, especially when the trauma has involved blows to the head.[30] On the other hand, in Latino cultures, where conceptions of "nerves" and the impact of nervous conditions on physical symptoms are commonplace, complaints referable to the nervous system—such "pseudoneurologic" problems as dizziness, numbness, weakness of extremities, and so forth—predictably would appear more frequently.[31] Cultural patterning of somatic symptoms also has become clear in ethnic groups such as Italians, Jews, Irish Catholics, and upper-middle-class white Europeans.[32] In these groups, culture appears to mediate severe trauma in producing somatic complaints of characteristic forms, rather than permitting a more frank breakdown in day-to-day psychosocial functioning.

In short, the mechanisms connecting trauma, culture, and somatoform symptoms appear to include several key elements. First, a narrative of terrible trauma is processed psychologically in different ways, depending on the sociocultural context (figure 5.1). The coherence versus incoherence of this narrative becomes a crucial feature in the transformation of traumatic events into somatoform symptoms. The sociocultural context patterns personal narrative at the psychological level, as well as the expression of narrative in social interactions, including those between patients and health care professionals. While the experience of overt psychological disturbance and breaking with customary roles may emerge as the patterned reaction to extreme stress in some cultures, elsewhere the transformation of terrible narrative into somatic symptoms may become the culturally sanctioned "way of knowing" and of processing such stress. Predictably,

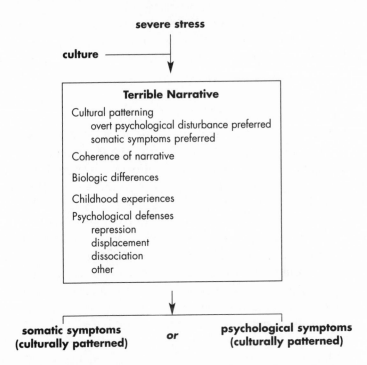

**FIGURE 5.1** *Schematic view of severe stress, culture, and narrative in somatoform symptoms.*

cultures vary not only in determining whether narratives of extreme stress express themselves by overt psychological disturbance as opposed to somatic symptoms, but also in the patterning of somatic symptoms when they occur.

At the individual level, one also expects variability in the reaction to extreme stress. Because of biological differences that are genetically determined, or because of varying childhood experiences that create greater or lesser vulnerability to trauma, some individuals may react to severe stress with less psychological disturbance or less somatic symptomatology. That is, within cultures, different biological characteristics or experiences may lead to individual variation in the processing of the terrible narrative. Therefore, not all individuals within a given culture react to traumatic stress in the same way, and culture influences the pattern by which individuals process their narratives of severe trauma. This variability may depend on the coherence versus incoherence of narrative structure, which links trauma, culture, and somatization.

## THE NEED FOR CHANGE

My colleagues and I have conducted a long-term project that aims to determine how war-related premigration experiences, changes in language, and acculturation are related to the presentation of somatoform symptoms in primary care. This study was designed to address gaps in existing knowledge about the links among severe trauma, PTSD, and somatization, and also about cultural differences in the clinical presentation of these problems. We have studied how Central American patients differ from other Latino and non-Latino patients in the expression of somatoform complaints, as well as the association between somatoform symptoms and PTSD among these patients. The research also focuses on the attitudes and behavioral responses of primary care physicians to these patients, and the extent to which barriers to access for health care and mental health services affect the presentation of somatoform symptoms.

In preliminary data from this research, we have confirmed cultural differences in the occurrence of somatization, as measured by the structured diagnostic instrument (CIDI). Specifically, among 1,456 subjects interviewed, we have found greater rates of somatization among Central American subjects (approximately 30 percent) than among other Latino (21 percent) and non-Latino (19 percent) comparison groups. Although we have observed high levels of traumatic stressors in the Central American group (72 percent), PTSD per se has not differed markedly from that affecting other Latinos and non-Latinos. This preliminary observation suggests that culture may mediate the link between severe stress and somatization, even without the development of PTSD, including its full manifestations of flashbacks, dreams, and related psychological phenomena. Our study represents only one of several that will yield new knowledge about mental health disorders among immigrant, refugee, and minority populations who seek primary care services.

In chapter 9, I spell out some implications of this work for changes in medical practice. The traumas experienced by many refugees, members of minority groups, and nonminority patients have created a new set of conditions and challenges for North American primary care and mental health providers. Much remains to be done in order to understand and heal the social, cultural, and political dimensions of trauma-related somatoform symptoms.

### ACKNOWLEDGMENT

I gratefully acknowledge the contributions of Rolando Castillo, Javier Escobar, Alison Holman, Holly Magaña, and Roxane Cohen Silver to the work described in this chapter.

# ◆ part three ◆

## STRUGGLES FOR HEALTH AND JUSTICE

# ◆ chapter six ◆

# Local Struggles for Access and Control

U NTIL POLICY MAKERS DECIDE on a coherent national program, practitioners and patients must continue to cope with difficulties of access, costs, and patient–doctor encounters at the local level. In communities throughout the United States, advocacy for the poor, minorities, immigrants, and refugees occurs in different forms and with varying success. Usually, such efforts involve coalitions that work toward changes in local policies. While informal networks of communication permit exchange of information about these activities, advocates seldom try to describe their efforts through publications. As a result, people who confront similar problems often do not learn about the achievements and failures of advocacy efforts in other localities.

Local advocacy occurs in many communities. For instance, activists in several geographic areas have worked together to stop "patient dumping" from private to public hospitals, yet publications on this problem have focused on research findings rather than successful or unsuccessful advocacy strategies.[1] Other groups have reported research on local barriers to access for indigent patients but have deemphasized the local or statewide advocacy efforts to which the research projects have been tied.[2] Concerned mainly about infant mortality, several local organizations have described their attempts to improve local access to prenatal and perinatal care, as well as other services for women and children.[3]

While still lacking a national policy that guarantees universal access, people in local communities throughout the United States will continue to face access barriers and will need to act locally in confronting this problem. In this chapter, I present the strategies that a countywide coalition used to improve access to services for the medically indigent during the mid-1980s to 1990s. These strategies focused on two issues: access to health care services for uninsured or underinsured people, and a proposed corporate takeover of a public university hospital that provided services disproportionately for the same people. While our work took place in a single county with some unique characteristics, I am presenting some details of these local actions, since similar advocacy techniques may prove useful in other localities as well. Although specific details of local policies and problems differ throughout the United States, the overall structures and processes of local decision making about access remain very similar. For that reason, the organizing strategies and experiences presented here may be applicable to similar problems elsewhere. After providing some background information about the county and about local health policies, I describe how our advocacy efforts emerged, as well as the strengths and weaknesses of local advocacy.

## LOCAL BACKGROUND

Orange County, California, has changed from a predominantly agricultural area to a center of industry, tourism, and entertainment. Minority groups constitute more than 25 percent of the county's more than 2 million residents; nearly 20 percent of the population is Latino. Hundreds of thousands of immigrants from a host of countries call Orange County home. Although known nationwide for its affluence, with a median family income of more than $46,000 per year, 10 percent of the county's families with children under five years of age earn incomes below the poverty line.[4] Local poverty remains largely hidden, since the county's busy freeways bypass the neighborhoods, parks, and barrios that hold an estimated 5,000 homeless persons and about 150,000 undocumented residents.

Major difficulties have arisen in health care for the poor in Orange County. Between 150,000 and 250,000 persons have lacked any medical insurance, public or private. About 76 percent of the uninsured in the county have comprised working people and their dependents; the workers have been based primarily in manufacturing, agriculture, landscaping, and service provision. Undocumented persons have constituted approximately 17 percent of the local uninsured population. The county's housing costs have ranked among the highest in the nation. Rent for a two-bedroom apartment has averaged about $800 per month, while the median price for a home reached $285,000.[5] A minimum wage earner's full-time monthly salary of about $730 has left little room for medical bills.

Several factors exacerbated the problems of Orange County's medically indigent. In 1975, the county sold its public hospital—the only public facility in the county—to the University of California, Irvine (UCI). As UCI Medical Center (UCIMC), the former county hospital continued to serve more than 60 percent of the indigent patients in the county. However, when federal, state, and county governments reduced funding for indigent care, UCIMC began to experience severe financial hardship. To help alleviate the financial difficulties, the hospital instituted a policy of up-front cash deposits. This policy restricted access to both inpatient and outpatient care.

Medi-Cal (California's Medicaid) "reforms" during the 1980s added to the problems of the poor in Orange County. First, the state implemented eligibility reductions mandated by new federal legislation governing Medicaid. In addition, the California legislature initiated major changes in the Medi-Cal program that included selective contracting to introduce price competition among hospitals, reduction of physician reimbursement, restriction of the "medically needy" provisions that allowed families to become eligible for benefits by deducting medical expenses from their incomes, cutbacks in covered services and medications, and increases in patients' required co-payments.

The new Medi-Cal laws also transferred responsibility for care of medically indigent adults from state to county governments, with only 70 percent of prior funding levels. Programs for medically indigent adults differed greatly among California counties. Orange County's Medically Indigent Adult (MIA) Program was one of the state's most restrictive. With a limited scope of services "to protect life, to prevent disability, and to prevent serious deterioration of health," MIA care was offered at contracting hospitals, at a few private clinics, and by those physicians who were willing to accept MIA reimbursement. Only U.S. citizens and documented residents were eligible for MIA.

Applicants to the MIA program faced a series of obstacles that impeded access to services. Initially, patients were required to submit extensive financial documentation during a seven- to eight-week waiting period for approval, often regardless of the severity of their illnesses. Moreover, MIA required the same large co-payments for the working poor as the Medi-Cal program. Its reimbursement rates were low and retrospective, leaving both providers and patients uncertain whether services would be covered. This uncertainty seriously restricted physician participation in the program. Because the program was not widely publicized in the community, many poor people did not know about it. Such limitations left thousands who previously had been covered by Medi-Cal in confusion and without access to care.

The county government's spending for indigent health care from its own funds also remained low. Despite its affluence, Orange County ranked at the bottom of the ten most populous California counties in per-capita expenditures on indigent health care, and 56th among all 58 California counties in overall per-capita health expenditures from local funds. The county operated no public hospital, administered no comprehensive-care clinic for anyone older than age five, and managed a state-funded MIA program to which the county's board of supervisors added no support from the county's general fund. These policies resulted in substantial barriers to access that affected uninsured low-income residents.

## COALITION BUILDING TO IMPROVE HEALTH CARE ACCESS

### *Origins of Advocacy Efforts*

During the mid-1980s, advocacy efforts began among a group of UCI faculty members, medical students, and residents who were facing severe problems in providing needed diagnostic and therapeutic services for indigent patients. Faculty reported these early cases in the medical literature soon after their occurrence.[6] In response to such concerns, medical students organized a large conference entitled "Health Care: A Right?" Presentations focused on the responsibility of the county and the university in health care provision and on problems in the MIA program.

The Orange County Task Force on Indigent Health Care convened to address issues that the conference had raised. Community providers concerned about indigent health care formed the core of this new coalition. Task-force membership included UCI faculty physicians, residents, and students; other health professionals; administrators of community clinics and hospitals; county employees; church people; and members of civic and social-service organizations, such as the Legal Aid Society and the League of Women Voters. The task force developed specific strategies to identify barriers to access and to advocate for reversal of these barriers.

As an organization, the task force consisted of a tightly knit nucleus of about 12 activists, who consistently attended monthly meetings and coordinated strategy, and a larger membership of approximately 50 individuals, who participate actively in response to initiatives from the leadership group. In addition to those above, the membership included health care professionals, concerned citizens, and consumers who faced difficulties with access. On an annual basis, members selected a chairperson, co-chairperson, and secretary. At least twice a year, members reviewed the task force's long- and short-term goals and evaluated progress toward meeting them.

Although only a minority of the UCI faculty became active in this work, task-force participants spanned the medical school's departments of medicine, pediatrics, obstetrics and gynecology, surgery, psychiatry, neurology, physical medicine and rehabilitation, and pathology, in addition to faculty in the social sciences and humanities on the university's general campus. From time to time, the actions of the task force led to opposition from some members of the university's administration and from other faculty who tried to limit UCI's involvement in indigent care because of the adverse impact that growing deficits exerted on teaching programs. On the other hand, such controversies did not restrict the ability of faculty, residents, and students to take part in the efforts of the task force to improve access to health care.

Members of the task force included participants from a wide range of service and educational agencies, but individual members did not formally represent those agencies in an official capacity. An early decision to work together as concerned individuals rather than as official representatives of other groups allowed the task force to adopt stronger advocacy positions and, at times, to use more confrontational tactics than the parent organizations would likely approve. On the other hand, task-force members' links with other organizations facilitated communication and coordination with other interested groups.

Whenever possible, task-force leaders also tried to coordinate advocacy efforts with prominent professional organizations and community agencies concerned with indigent care. For instance, the officers and staff of the Orange County Medical Association and the Hospital Council of Southern California cooperated with the task force in presenting testimony on indigent care in public hearings at the county and state levels. Similarly, the United Way of Orange County sought assistance from the task force in preparing a report on barriers to access and in advocating policy changes from the county government. In these instances, the task force's official independence allowed cooperation among organizations while maintaining a formal separation of their policy positions.

In early meetings, task-force members developed a conceptual approach to strategy that emphasized three components. First, research was required to document local barriers to access and the failures of current policies. Second, political work targeting both the county government and local health care institutions was necessary to improve access; research findings about access problems predictably would help guide these political efforts. Third, legal advocacy was needed to strengthen the impact of political organizing on local policy. Strengths and weaknesses became clear in each of these three arenas of strategy.

### Research Strategies

*Research to document local access problems.* The research strategies of the task force aimed to raise the consciousness of county residents about indigent care problems and buttress political strategies that targeted policies of county government and health care institutions. Initially, task-force members interviewed and documented the severity of medical problems among 200 Orange County residents who could not receive services due to lack of cash deposit, private insurance, and government coverage.[7] In a consensus review by practicing physicians, the investigators found that 60 percent of the study's subjects had a moderate-to-high likelihood of long-term disability, and that 79 percent had diseases for which medical services were judged to have a moderate-to-curative impact if they were available. Diagnoses in these persons included pregnancy, epilepsy, multiple sclerosis, diabetes mellitus, serious heart disease, and cancer. Persons with more serious illnesses were less likely to obtain care than those with milder problems.

Second, the researchers examined financial barriers to care among those persons already within the academic medica center system.[8] This study assessed patients who received care at a UCI-affiliated outpatient clinic during a six-week period. Using a questionnaire completed by clinic physicians at the time of each patient visit, the study documented that 94 patients, or nearly 5 percent of the clinic's patient load, were unable to receive diagnostic and/or therapeutic services due to financial barriers. Unaffordable services included consultations, radiological and ultrasound studies, medication, and surgery. These patients manifested a wide range of medical problems, such as hearing loss, congestive heart failure, seizure disorders, and psychiatric disturbances. Findings from this study dramatized that financial barriers interfered with provision of appropriate medical services, even among persons who could gain access to primary care.

Third, the task force researchers continued their work when they received a grant from a foundation affiliated with a private Catholic hospital for a needs assessment of the indigent population in the hospital's catchment area.[9] This study attempted to implement several principles of community-oriented primary care and small-area analysis, as described in chapter 2. A population-based survey showed that the poor of northern Orange County reported problems with access to care more often than a comparable group of the poor nationwide. The survey also found that this local group was approximately three times as likely to lack health insurance as the national average. Low utilization of preventive services, such as prenatal care, immunizations, or pap smears, was especially striking. In response to this research, the sponsoring hospital initiated programs designed to meet some of these needs.

Two additional studies of Orange County's health care system further highlighted the access problems faced by the poor. In one study, spearheaded by a task force member, the League of Women Voters interviewed officials at local health care institutions and identified problems with the MIA program, the need for additional county-funded prenatal care, and a lack of sufficient services for indigent children. The study spawned several league-sponsored forums that presented public concerns to county officials and health care providers. In another study based on in-depth interviews with providers and consumers, the newly formed United Way Health Care Task Force, a broad coalition of health providers, insurers, businesses, labor representatives, county government staff, social service agencies, and health advocates, published a report entitled *Orange County—Health Care Crisis*, which received wide distribution. Warning about the "critical condition of health care services," the report offered a comprehensive analysis of the current health care problems facing the county.

## Political Strategies

Buttressed by research, political action for policy change became the task force's principal activity. Advocacy by the task force aimed primarily to change policies at the county level and increase access at local health care institutions. Task force members also participated in advocacy and legislative efforts on the state and national levels.

*Targeting county government.* The task force's political pressure on the county government began with a series of private meetings. Centering on the problems of funding, eligibility, and access in the MIA program, these efforts included meetings between task force members and MIA staff, aides to the board of supervisors, the director of the Orange County Health Care Agency, and the county's administrative officer. At these meetings, task force researchers presented findings from the studies described above, as well as case reports that documented the adverse impact of financial barriers to care. Although county officials asserted that no additional funds were available, these early meetings established a dialogue that later led to improved access.

Specific areas of progress included new sites of service and streamlined eligibility processing. Task force representatives joined with members of the Orange County Coalition of Free and Community Clinics in a monthly meeting with the county's MIA staff. Participants lobbied successfully for the inclusion of additional clinics as contractual MIA providers. The county also substituted a form of declarative eligibility in place of the original process of extensive and unwieldy eligibility documentation. As a result, access to MIA coverage improved substantially, with a more than 300-percent increase in the number of approved applications, and a 140-percent rise in the number of claims that the MIA program paid.

With the county's failure to increase MIA funding or scope of services, the task force began a series of presentations and funding requests at the county budget hearings held annually by the board of supervisors in early summer. Within the hearings, the task force sought funds for community clinics that served persons without support from MIA, Medi-Cal, and other county health programs. This strategy aimed to raise public awareness about problems of the medically indigent and add momentum for reform.

The task force's testimony and press releases led to extensive publicity, including a highly publicized confrontation at a budget hearing between task force members and county supervisors. Although the budget hearings initially resulted in no additional funding, the board of supervisors commissioned an investigation of health care for the poor. During the following year, a coalition of task force members and representatives from other organizations concerned about health care access successfully lobbied the board of supervisors and the Orange County Health Care Agency staff for expansion of county-funded prenatal care. With the hiring of additional nurse practitioners, 500 additional prenatal positions were added, an increase of one-third.

The same coalition took action when the state made available a block grant to counties in place of increasing state funding for indigent health care. This one-time grant of $6.1 million to Orange County carried no requirements concerning its expenditure. County officials proposed using only about $1 million of the grant for health care, and the rest primarily to raise salaries of county employees. Extensive lobbying coordinated by the chairman of the United Way Health Care Task Force, as well as participation by the Orange County Medical Association and the Hospital Council of Southern California, led to an approval of $4 million for health services and staff, plus the first county grant of $300,000 to community clinics for general medical services.

*Targeting health care institutions.* Because UCIMC was the largest provider of health services for the poor in Orange County, policy decisions that reduced public funding for indigent care disproportionately affected this medical center. Facing multimillion-dollar deficits caused in large part by low levels of reimbursement, UCIMC had initiated various administrative procedures that created financial barriers to care. The task force carried out a multifaceted strategy to reduce these barriers.

Task force members frequently brought to the attention of UCIMC administrators specific patients who could not receive care at UCIMC due to the up-front deposit policy. Further, the research projects described above revealed that many other patients either could not gain access to the medical center or, if they did gain access, could not obtain needed diagnostic or therapeutic services because of financial barriers. In response to this input, UCIMC administrators developed a protocol by which, at the request of faculty or residents, the up-front deposit could be waived and teaching funds used for diagnostic or therapeutic procedures. As acknowledged by UCIMC officials, waiver of the deposit in specific instances became an alternative mode of access for indigent patients who happened to encounter community advocates. Though clearly not eliminating barriers to access, these policy changes improved the problems that the task force's research revealed at the academic medical center.

An attempt to sell or lease UCIMC to a for-profit hospital chain also became a focus for political organizing by the task force. Because of its chronic financial crisis, UCIMC negotiated with several for-profit corporations that expressed interest in buying or managing the hospital. When these corporations did not ensure that they would provide continuing access for publicly insured or uninsured patients, the task force helped organize a broad coalition that opposed corporate takeover. The central administration of the University of California acknowledged the impact of this opposition when it eventually decided to continue its own management of the hospital, without direct corporate involvement. More details about this struggle appear later in this chapter.

Task force members also participated in efforts to keep open UCIMC's two satellite outpatient clinics and its pediatric clinic. Each year, UCIMC administrators developed plans either to close the satellite clinics as a cost-saving measure or to institute mandatory deposit policies that would seriously hinder access. Responding to pressures from a community coalition coordinated by the task force, university officials reversed proposals for new cutbacks and financial barriers. Moreover, plans to close the pediatric clinic at UCIMC and move it to a nearby private children's hospital met with the task force's efforts to ensure that these changes did not affect the access of indigent children to needed services. In private meetings and in response to adverse publicity, university officials decided to defer these alterations in the organization of pediatric care.

Efforts by task force members contributed to policy changes at other health care institutions in addition to UCIMC. Participants cooperated with a network of private Catholic hospitals in developing new programs to expand services to indigent patients. Task force members also worked for greater compliance by private hospitals with the access requirements of Medi-Cal and MIA contracts. Further, task force participants helped reduce the problem of dumping unstable patients from private emergency departments to UCIMC and its satellite clinics by helping patients who experienced dumping file legal complaints.

*State and national efforts.* In addition to local work, the task force participated in complementary state and national advocacy efforts. On several occasions, task force members and their medically indigent clients received invitations to give testimony before the state legislature's Committee on Medi-Cal Oversight. This committee investigated problems created by the transfer of responsibility for medically indigent adults to the counties and explored problems of service restriction linked to further proposed Medi-Cal cutbacks. Task force leaders testified at state hearings in support of a tougher antidumping law. Members took part in efforts for a state health plan to improve access. At the national level, task force leaders testified on health policy before committees of Congress and worked with professional groups advocating a national health program.

*Strengths and weaknesses of the political strategies.* An important contribution has involved the sensitization of political and health care institutions to the task force's oversight. In particular, officials of the county government recognized that further cutbacks or administrative barriers to care would meet with consistent public attention and opposition from a coalition of interested individuals and groups. Likewise, administrators of the academic medical center and private hospitals realized that their own policies on indigent care continued to receive critical scrutiny. In such examples, the task force gained recognition as an organization legitimately advocating for the medically indigent.

On the other hand, this strategy remained basically defensive and incremental. Task force members devoted substantial time and energy to documenting financial barriers to care and to working for policy changes in county government and health care institutions. For most task force participants, these advocacy efforts were voluntary activities, outside their usual jobs. Such activities became difficult to sustain when each year brought new threats of cutbacks or other barriers to access. Further, efforts to maintain services at a minimum level did not lead to more creative and proactive programs that would improve the overall organization and provision of care. The defensive nature of these advocacy strategies became perhaps their most discouraging feature.

### Legal Strategies

The task force's strategies for change have included a limited focus on legal action, which generally remained subordinate to the research and political strategies. Task force members encountered medically indigent clients whose treatment by county officials or private providers seemed to fall outside the bounds of law. County policies, such as denying MIA coverage to the undocumented and the lack of required notices in contracting hospitals about MIA benefits, resulted in unavailability of needed care. In other California counties, litigation led to reform and expansion of county indigent health services.

Task force membership included attorneys working with local law centers that represented indigent clients. These legal professionals initiated actions for individual patients who faced financial barriers to care and testified to the county board of supervisors in public hearings regarding the county's lack of legal compliance in its health programs with federal and state standards. Casework involved patients who could not gain MIA or Medi-Cal eligibility because of faulty administrative procedures and persons with MIA coverage who could not receive covered medical or dental services at local contracting hospitals. With legal advocacy, court litigation in these cases usually did not prove necessary. Further, coordination of initiatives between the task force and local law centers heightened the attention that such advocacy efforts received from county officials and administrators of health care institutions.

Legal efforts by the task force led to a major policy change concerning patients legalized under the national Immigration Reform and Control Act ("amnesty program"). The state Medi-Cal program offered only "restricted" coverage for emergency and pregnancy-related care to adult amnesty recipients; the county generally provided no additional services through MIA or other programs for nonemergency conditions. A task force attorney and paralegal worker presented to county officials the case of an immigrant woman approved under the amnesty program who experienced recurrent episodes of acute and chronic cholecystitis. Despite documented gallstones for which consulting surgeons recommended cholecystectomy, local hospitals would not admit her because they did not consider her condition an emergency and because the county would not extend MIA coverage. As a result of legal advocacy concerning this case, the county accepted responsibility to provide needed nonemergency care to immigrants who received amnesty. Adult amnesty recipients with restricted Medi-Cal thus became eligible for MIA, a change that made health care available to thousands of immigrants in the county.

Several task force members also played a key role in the formation and funding of the county's first public interest law project. This project hired a lawyer to focus on impact litigation in health care. Task force members assisted in gathering a series of cases for legal action.

In some areas, such as care for undocumented patients who did not qualify for the amnesty program, difficult problems persisted that could not be addressed without litigation. Although limited federal and state funds became available for services to individuals who gained approval for amnesty, other undocumented residents remained uncovered. The California counties varied widely in health care expenditures for this group, and Orange County recognized no financial responsibility for services to the undocumented beyond a small fund set up for emergency care at UCIMC, which actually covered only a fraction of the care provided annually. Because litigation in this area would prove a complex undertaking, a shortage of staff time and resources prohibited local agencies from formally taking legal action. Locating suitable plaintiffs, such as undocumented clients with severe illnesses who did not receive services due to immigration status and who were willing to risk deportation for the sake of litigation, also became an ethical and practical dilemma.

The new public interest law firm also initiated a legal project focusing on the MIA program. When the county's reimbursement rate for the MIA program dropped to an average of five cents on the dollar of billed charges, fewer private hospitals were willing to care for uninsured or publicly insured patients, and the county medical association reported that only 7 percent of member physicians were willing to accept a patient with MIA coverage.

Plans for the MIA project called for follow-up to research done by the task force's team. The project's research assistant, with guidance from the research group and lawyers at both the Public Law Center of Orange County (PLC) and the Legal Aid Society of Orange County (LAS), worked to identify patients who experienced barriers to access under the county's MIA program. The Poverty and Race Research Action Council of Washington, D.C., awarded a seed grant of $10,000 for the project. PLC and LAS provided continuing support by assigning lawyers and paralegals to work on access barriers.

The first challenge facing the project was a paucity of information about the MIA program. Project staff identified and obtained copies of the MIA provider manual, the sporadically published MIA bulletins, and the MIA contract signed by the participating providers. However, no clear published regulations were found specifying how the fiscal intermediary and the medical review board made decisions about coverage. In addition, it was discovered that the MIA Hotline, a special telephone number for patients and providers to inquire about the program and obtain tentative answers to coverage questions, was consistently busy during business hours. One staff member called the number thirteen times during a four-week period before she was able to talk with someone at MIA.

The research assistant introduced the project to the medical community by meeting with caseworkers at community clinics and hospitals with large MIA constituencies. She talked with them about the goal of helping prospective MIA patients through the application process and with any problems that they might subsequently encounter. Several of these providers referred appropriate MIA patients to the project.

As a result of this work, six broad barriers to access were identified: cumbersome eligibility processing, including extensive paperwork, delays in approval, and a small number of application sites; excessive waiting times for needed medical services; burdensome patient co-payments and deposit policies; a narrow range of medical services provided; language and cultural barriers; and small numbers of participating providers.

In an effort to remove barriers to access, the project developed several strategies. With the purpose of educating newcomers to the area of health law in Orange County, the project collected information about the MIA program and prepared a memorandum that outlined its history and some of its problems. The project also assembled a packet of documents to be used by advocates. Those materials included a short reporting form for providers, a more detailed questionnaire in English and Spanish for patients (which complemented ongoing local research on access), a demand letter, a model legal brief, a research memorandum regarding the procedure for bringing a civil writ, and two research memoranda discussing substantive bases to challenge health care access barriers. A descriptive list of typical clients helped by the project, with a description of their problems and interventions on their behalf, was also prepared.

Equipped with that information, advocates were able to accept cases, analyze them, and resolve them either informally or through litigation. PLC maintained a database of lawyers and paralegal workers in Orange County who accepted *pro bono* cases or were willing to do so. In the area of health care access and payment disputes, PLC coordinated approximately 40 volunteer attorneys to assist clients with the problems identified by the project. Nearly 10 percent of PLC's work came to involve health access issues.

When a patient was identified, LAS or PLC found an attorney or paralegal willing to accept the case, prepared a brief summary of the facts of the case, and sent that information along with any necessary forms to the attorney or paralegal. The attorney or paralegal then handled the case, at no cost to the client, until the access problem was resolved.

Clients accepted by PLC were placed on a priority basis. These priorities were decided on the basis of medical urgency and estimated numbers of patients affected by the specific barriers in the MIA program to be overcome. As concrete barriers were targeted, individual cases were analyzed to determine whether they fulfilled the criteria necessary to challenge each barrier successfully. Although the project emphasized access to county-funded health care, providers made inquiries to clarify both MIA and Medi-Cal eligibility issues. Skill in identification of the access problem and the correct administrative level to take action, as well as knowledge of referral agencies, developed through assistance to the patients referred.

Several inquiries involved complicated issues of immigrant eligibility. In one case, a cancer patient needing surgery had been wrongly identified in the Medi-Cal program as eligible for only emergency services because of improper identification of her immigration status. The legal advocate was able to secure full coverage Medi-Cal by correct identification of the patient's immigration category.

Scope of coverage in the MIA program was an issue in a larger number of cases, including coverage of hernia surgery and prescription drugs. Advocacy resulted in receipt of needed services without court action. Legal advocacy also led to changes in several county eligibility regulations governing the MIA program.

Staff time committed to the project was not extensive. Specifically, one lawyer at LAS spent about 5-percent effort (of his total workload) on the project, at a total annual cost of about

$3,200. The estimated in-kind costs of *pro bono* legal professionals who donated their services were hard to estimate, but PLC cases averaged approximately 15.6 hours of legal assistance time. These *pro bono* services would be valued at approximately $2,730 per case. Reliance on *pro bono* legal advocacy substantially reduced the cost per client assisted by private counsel to about $394.

The project also facilitated working relations with county officials, who often were unaware of the barriers to access that emerged. In response to legal advocacy, caseworkers for the county became more cooperative in responding to access barriers through changes in administrative procedures.

Local advocates viewed the project as a necessary step in a larger strategy to improve access to health care.[10] Project participants hoped that the packet of research methods, instruments, and legal documents would prove useful for other advocates around the country. After advocates learned the requirements, goals, and problems of public insurance programs like MIA, they could challenge government agencies, health care providers, and policy makers to make such programs more efficient and responsive. More importantly, advocates could work to make the process of obtaining health care more manageable and less degrading for clients.

It is likely that local projects will become increasingly needed because of trends that reinforce the role of county governments and managed care in policy decisions about health care access. Policy decisions have emphasized greater decentralization of policy and funding decisions regarding health care to county governments. Such trends are likely to persist, especially if national health reform proposals do not create uniform standards of access throughout the country. Adoption of any national health reform proposal, if co-payments and exclusions remain, is likely to leave substantial barriers to access intact. Local variability in access will persist, especially in areas where county governments have not assumed a commitment to delivering services for the medically needy.

## ORGANIZING TO RESIST CORPORATE TAKEOVER

The involvement of for-profit corporations in public hospitals has stimulated debate. Critics have pointed out a series of potential problems with the corporate management of such centers, including ethical problems, financial difficulties, conflicts between corporate and academic goals, and limits on services to indigent patients. Supporters have argued that negotiations between academic medical centers and corporations can resolve such issues.[11]

Since the mid-1980s, the University of California periodically has considered the corporate takeover of state teaching hospitals that have experienced financial hardship. These hospitals have included especially those institutions that previously were owned and operated by local county governments but that were later purchased by the university to help support its teaching and research programs. Consideration of corporate takeover focused mainly on the most financially troubled teaching hospital in the university system: UCIMC. After extensive discussion, the university administration decided not to accept corporate management or ownership. The prospect of a corporate takeover at this public university hospital met with broad opposition at the local, state, and national levels.[12]

### *The Option of Corporate Management at a University Medical Center*

UCIMC was the former county hospital of Orange County. When the California College of Medicine moved from Los Angeles to Irvine in 1968, it began to use the county hospital as its main teaching facility. To consolidate the role of the hospital as an academic institution, the University of California purchased the hospital from the county in 1976. The county government continued to contract with UCIMC for services that remained the legal responsibility of the county: certain emergency services, the treatment of custody patients, and the care of some indigent patients without medical insurance. In absolute dollars, these county contracts remained at approximately the same level, about $10 million annually, during the next decade; adjusted for inflation, the county's financial contribution to UCIMC during this period actually declined.

Orange County's per-capita spending on medical care for indigent patients remained the lowest among the ten most populous California counties. For example, San Francisco County paid approximately ten times more funds per capita for health care for indigent patients than Orange County. Because UCIMC and its satellite community clinics provided care to the majority of indigent patients in the county, the low level of county support created severe financial problems for the institution.

UCIMC also was vulnerable to changes in state and federal reimbursement policies. This hospital maintained one of the highest proportions of indigent patients—approximately 60 percent (or 70 percent when indigent Medicare patients were included)—among university hospitals in the United States that did not operate under the auspices of municipal or county governments. After the state's Medicaid system began a system of prospective reimbursement for inpatient care, UCIMC served Medicaid patients at a daily reimbursement rate that was markedly lower than the actual costs to the institution. Diagnosis-related groups under Medicare, which provided reimbursement based on patients' diagnoses, heightened UCIMC's financial problems. As in other hospitals that served a high proportion of poor people, the indigent Medicare patients treated at UCIMC tended to be sicker, were more apt to have several diseases at a higher level of severity, and were harder to place after discharge than nonindigent elderly patients. These factors made it more difficult to cover the costs of hospitalization through the reimbursement allowed by Medicare.

Under these circumstances, the financial condition of UCIMC became chronically bleak. The hospital faced annual operating deficits of approximately $9 million. Additionally, UCIMC's physical plant was deteriorating. Funds for major capital expenditures were not immediately forthcoming from the state or county. The university's board of regents, which held financial responsibility for the entire University of California system, expressed concern about deficit financing at any of the university hospitals. Administrators set a high priority on the consideration of options that would improve UCIMC's financial condition.

Against this background, the prospect of a corporate solution seemed attractive. Officials at UCI entered into discussions with a number of for-profit health care chains concerning the sale or management of UCIMC. University administrators and faculty members visited academic medical centers that had been taken over by corporations elsewhere in the country. A committee of administrators and faculty members recommended that as a model for discussions with corporations, UCIMC should use a preliminary agreement negotiated between American Medical International (AMI)—a for-profit hospital chain based in Beverly Hills, California—and George Washington University Hospital. The administration at UCI then entered into negotiations with AMI, with the goal of corporate management of UCIMC.

AMI had focused on the purchase or management of academic medical centers in several regions of the United States. These centers, according to the corporation's strategy, would function as "flagships," providing prestigious university affiliations and serving as referral centers for regional networks of clinics and hospitals owned or managed by AMI. Affiliations with academic medical centers could offer AMI substantial advantages in public relations and also promote the vertical integration of corporate facilities within particular regions. After AMI reached an agreement on affiliation with Creighton University in Omaha, Nebraska, the corporation engaged in negotiations with George Washington University Hospital and academic medical centers in other regions with the aim of setting up similar arrangements. Penetrating the lucrative Southern California market was a highly desirable objective for AMI. From this perspective, its investment in UCIMC could enhance the development and integration of a regional health care system.

### A New Private Hospital

Within Orange County, AMI also hoped to profit from a new private hospital to be built in the city of Irvine. UCIMC was located in the central part of Orange County, where most of the county's indigent and minority residents lived. Irvine, which was closer to the coast, was the fastest growing city in California and attracted a wealthy population. The city of Irvine included the main UCI campus, as well as the basic science departments of the College of Medicine.

A conflict previously had arisen between the College of Medicine and other local interest groups about a new hospital in Irvine. Administrators and faculty members of the College of Medicine favored the construction of the facility on the university campus. This hospital, they argued, would then become a second major academic medical center that would serve the university's goals of teaching, research, and clinical practice. Moreover, a campus-based hospital would attract a higher proportion of insured patients, who could contribute positively to the financial situation of the College of Medicine. Opposition to an on-campus site for the hospital came from private practitioners and others in the Irvine area who feared competition from a campus-based hospital. Several local corporations, including the Irvine Company, the major land-development corporation in southern Orange County, opposed the on-campus site. These corporations hoped to create a biotechnology center adjacent to the new hospital on land owned by the Irvine Company—land unsuitable for development of housing because of its proximity to a military air station.

The resolution of this controversy eventually favored the off-campus site, but with a strong role for the university. In awarding a certificate of need to permit construction at the off-campus location, the state government required the coalition to negotiate an affiliation agreement with the College of Medicine and to include a representative of the university on the new hospital's board of directors. Subsequently, the off-campus coalition began to search for financing to cover construction costs. After several possible financing schemes failed, the coalition faced a possible default on the deadline for breaking ground specified by the certificate of need.

Under these circumstances, the coalition found a sympathetic ear at AMI. After brief negotiations involving AMI officials, leaders of the off-campus coalition, and university administrators, AMI agreed to finance the construction of the new hospital and later to manage it as part of its Southern California network. UCI accepted an affiliation that included membership on the new hospital's governing board.

The involvement of AMI with the university therefore had two parts. First, AMI was to construct, own, and manage a new private hospital in the city of Irvine. The hospital would be physically separate from the university campus but closely affiliated with the College of Medicine.

Second, AMI would negotiate a lease-management contract with UCIMC. Under this contract, AMI would assume responsibility for UCIMC's operating deficit and give the university several million dollars per year in return for the lease. AMI would also commit substantial funds for capital improvements at UCIMC. Although workers at UCIMC would become employees of AMI, faculty members would continue to work for the university, and AMI would provide faculty salary support similar in amount to what the university previously received from the hospital. The College of Medicine would make decisions about academic policy, but UCIMC's governing board would include representatives from both AMI and the university. AMI would also promise to provide care to indigent patients under existing contracts with county, state, and federal agencies. However, AMI's future intentions about renewing these contracts, as well as the fate of uninsured patients, remained to be determined.

### Resistance to Corporate Management

The plans for corporate management of UCIMC generated opposition from organized labor, university faculty members, California legislators, officials of other University of California medical centers, local private hospitals, officials of the county government, and the university's central administration.

*Unionized workers.* Among all affected groups, UCIMC employees stood to lose the most from corporate management. Workers at the medical center had won bargaining rights with the university through earlier union elections. A national union—the American Federation of State, County, and Municipal Employees (AFSCME)—represented the majority of UCIMC workers. The union had improved wages and benefits through contracts negotiated with the University of California. These obligations required that UCIMC increase wages and benefits as required by the University of California system, despite the hospital's vulnerable financial condition.

Corporate takeover fundamentally would have changed UCIMC's relation with its employees. With the exception of faculty members and a small number of other professionals, UCIMC workers would become employees of the corporation that managed the medical center. Although the draft of the agreement with AMI called for a grace period of about one year before employees could be fired without cause, the corporation's previous record indicated that reductions in staff would probably be a major cost-cutting tactic after the corporate takeover. Agreements about employees' seniority, salaries, and benefits that previously had been negotiated by the University of California and AFSCME might also be retracted. Perhaps most important, AFSCME's right to remain the legal bargaining agent for UCIMC employees under corporate management was in doubt. The union was also worried that corporate management at a major state-supported teaching hospital would set a precedent for similar takeovers at institutions throughout the country. Moreover, in its policy positions, the union argued that the future survival of publicly supported hospitals depended largely on their continuing to serve as providers of last resort, and that corporate management threatened these hospitals' services to indigent patients.

Faced with these concerns, AFSCME mounted a national campaign to block corporate management at UCIMC. The union's national office in Washington, D.C., allocated funds and staff time to this goal. Its department of public policy prepared detailed criticisms of the lease-management proposal. AFSCME's staff lobbied vigorously with the central administration of the University of California in Berkeley and with key state legislators in Sacramento.

*University of California faculty members.* The financial problems of UCIMC had affected university faculty members adversely in several ways. The salaries of many physicians on the faculty were derived in large part from hospital revenues.

Because of UCIMC's deficit, funding for contracted physician services had been frozen or reduced. The hospital also provided much of the support for the faculty members' private practices and clinical-research activities; UCIMC's difficulties had led to layoffs of staff members and cutbacks in laboratory, radiology, social work, nutrition, and other support services. These changes created inconveniences for faculty members in their teaching, research, and practice. The hospital's fiscal crisis increased the administrative workload of the faculty; faculty members were needed to restructure clinical services, make decisions about reductions in staffing, and assume other responsibilities. Burdened by such difficulties, most medical faculty members supported the efforts of campus administrators to negotiate a corporate management contract.

An active minority of the faculty, however, opposed corporate management. These faculty members circulated critical analyses of the AMI proposal in particular, and of corporate involvement at university hospitals in general. Their criticism focused on ethical issues, the unclear economic implications of the proposed corporate takeover, AMI's previous record, potential conflicts between AMI and UCIMC's educational and research goals and clinical practice priorities, and the impact of the takeover on indigent patients. These faculty members also prepared an alternative proposal that called for increased public support for UCIMC, stronger management at the center, and a larger proportion of insured patients. Faculty members raised these concerns in committees, at faculty meetings, and in interviews requested by the press and by state legislators. A loose coalition of faculty members, students, and union leaders met regularly to coordinate strategy. This group also collaborated with the county-wide Task Force on Indigent Health Care.

An important issue considered by the faculty as a whole was the economic health of AMI and similar corporations. AMI's business operations had been profitable for several years. Analysts of for-profit hospital corporations had long predicted, however, that such earnings would cease to grow. Such corporations had depended on debt financing for capital expenses. They had also encouraged the use of expensive diagnostic and therapeutic procedures, encouraged lengthy hospitalization and surgery for insured patients, and reduced costs by laying off employees and using temporary or part-time workers. Predictably, the cost-containment strategies adopted by public- and private-insurance programs would interfere with the corporations' ability to sustain high profit margins through such strategies. Utilization review procedures, prospective reimbursement, required second opinions, and similar measures would limit the profits available to the chains.

Partly because of such cost-containment efforts, the profits of AMI and similar firms started to dwindle. As the occupancy rates at AMI hospitals declined, the company announced a drop in net income. After this announcement, the market value of AMI stocks fell rapidly, with parallel declines in the value of the stocks of other for-profit hospital chains. Subsequently, AMI continued to report declining income. In short, the long-term economic health of AMI and the rest of the for-profit hospital industry became uncertain. This change in AMI's financial prospects emerged as a critical consideration in the faculty's decision-making process.

Because of the concerns raised by faculty members, the faculty senate of the College of Medicine, the faculty's formal policy-making body, considered in detail the opposing view of corporate management. Although the senate voted to support continuing negotiations with AMI, it also requested that any agreement reached between the University of California and AMI be returned to the faculty for final approval. Moreover, the senate voted to establish a new committee to study alternatives to corporate management.

*The California legislature.* The prospect of a corporate takeover at a University of California teaching hospital generated intense interest among state legislators. During the early 1970s, the legislature had supported the university's purchase of county hospitals in Orange, Sacramento, and San Diego Counties. In doing so, the legislature had tried to improve the teaching programs of the University of California medical schools at Irvine, Davis, and San Diego, while providing a reliable source of health care for indigent patients. The negotiations between UCI and AMI raised concerns about state support for a teach-

ing institution that would contribute to the profits of a multinational corporation. Legislators addressed a variety of legal
and ethical issues, including the hospital's status as a tax-sup-
ported state institution, the care of the poor, the effect of corporate management on educational goals, and the relation of state
funds to corporate profits.

In particular, legislators focused on the use of clinical teaching support funds and additional funds to cover operating
deficits that the legislature had allocated to the University of
California medical schools and teaching hospitals. Under the
draft agreement between UCIMC and AMI, the university
would channel these funds to the corporation; in return, AMI
would take responsibility for the hospital's deficit. The clinical
teaching funds allocated to UCIMC totaled more than $8.3 mil-
lion annually. Some legislators worried that this money would
constitute an inappropriate public subsidy to a private corporation. They pointed out the earnings of AMI's top executives
(its chairman earned more than several million dollars annually in salary and stock options) and asked whether further
support in the form of educational funds was justifiable. Without the clinical teaching allocation, AMI officials noted, a lease-
management agreement would not be feasible.

*Other University of California teaching hospitals.* The chancel-
lors and hospital administrators at the University of California
campuses in Los Angeles and San Francisco opposed the takeover proposal. These hospitals were historically the strongest in
the university system. Both institutions continued to be financially successful, despite changes in patterns of public funding.
The proportion of insured patients remained higher at the Los
Angeles and San Francisco hospitals than at the Irvine, Davis,
and San Diego facilities, all of which were former county hospitals. Furthermore, there had been no attempts to redistribute
economic resources from the stronger to the poorer University
of California hospitals. Despite the university regents' ultimate
responsibility for the five university hospitals, a tradition of
financial independence had generally permitted each hospital
to be operated independently.

The Los Angeles and San Francisco hospitals did not support

the proposed management of the center by a for-profit corporation. Administrators at the University of California at Los Angeles and San Francisco continued to favor state university
administration for the center. They questioned whether corporate management would strive to fulfill the educational and
service objectives of a public teaching hospital. Similarly, the
precedent that would be set by the UCIMC agreement might
lead to similar takeover attempts at Davis or San Diego. The possibility that the five University of California hospitals might be
administered quite differently was troubling to officials at the
Los Angeles and San Francisco institutions. They communicated
their opposition to the university president's office in Berkeley.

*Local private hospitals and county government.* UCIMC's negotiations with a for-profit corporation did not gain support in
the surrounding community. Local private hospitals feared
new competition from UCIMC. Staff members at nearby private hospitals expressed concern that the university's prestige
and resources might give unfair advantages to AMI. These clinicians also objected to the transfer of tax-generated public
funds directly to a private, for-profit corporation. When the
officials of a major children's hospital in Orange County
decided to end the affiliation of some of its teaching programs
with the university, they cited concerns about corporate management at UCIMC as the reason.

The county government did not look favorably on the AMI
proposal either. Although Orange County had provided low
levels of support to UCIMC, county supervisors and administrators still sought to maintain control over the programs that
the county did fund. County officials expressed skepticism that
a for-profit corporation would manage these programs appro-
priately. During the negotiations with AMI, county supervisors
decided not to renew a contract with UCIMC to operate a radio
base station in the county's trauma system. Supervisors cited
uncertainty about the AMI proposal as a major factor in the
decision to discontinue this important contract.

*The central administration of the University of California.* After
encouraging exploration of the possibility of corporate management, the central administration of the university received nega-

tive reactions to AMI's proposal. The union representing UCIMC employees, concerned legislators, and officials of other University of California hospitals had all voiced concern. The university's attorneys examined the proposal and pointed out serious legal problems without simple solutions—in particular, the fact that the contracts that the university had previously signed with the union could not be transferred to a private corporation. Also, a potential legal problem was the proposed transfer to AMI of public funds allocated by the legislature for medical education. These political and legal considerations swayed the university administration against the agreement with AMI.

### Deciding Against the Corporate Option

Ultimately, the central administration of the University of California decided not to support the proposal for corporate lease-management at UCIMC. In making this decision, the university's administration committed itself to maintaining direct authority over the operations of all five university hospitals. By rejecting corporate management, administrators also implied that they would pursue efforts to resolve UCIMC's financial difficulties.

Even before the decision was announced, the university moved to obtain additional funding for UCIMC from the state government. In its budget proposals to the state legislature, the university asked for funds to cover operational deficits or other short-term needs at the three financially troubled University of California teaching hospitals at Irvine, Davis, and San Diego. UCIMC received the largest share of these funds. In addition, proposals for capital improvements at UCIMC were passed. These financial measures reaffirmed the state government's continuing commitment to support UCIMC.

Austerity measures and tight budgeting at UCIMC also improved its financial situation. A freeze on hiring new employees, more efficient accounting procedures, and efforts to increase the proportion of insured patients at the hospital led to a reduction in the operating deficit. Meanwhile, UCI administrators and faculty members continued to negotiate with AMI about the university's role in the new hospital that was constructed in Irvine. Officials of both AMI and the university stated publicly that the hospital would undertake mainly community service and primary care, whereas UCIMC would continue to function mainly as a teaching hospital offering tertiary care. Skeptics inside and outside the university predicted and later confirmed that the private hospital in Irvine would become a more specialized and technologically oriented institution, which ultimately competed with UCIMC for insured patients and financial resources. Therefore, although the university decided against AMI's management of UCIMC, the corporation remained active in the local marketplace.

Nonetheless, the University of California's rejection of corporate management at UCIMC set an important precedent. The increasing involvement of for-profit hospital chains in academic medical centers remained a trend in health care throughout the 1990s. For instance, mergers frequently occurred with participation by for-profit corporations, especially in cities like New York, Boston, Chicago, and San Francisco. The recurrent crises of the University of California hospitals persisted. Lacking a national health program, medical centers will continue to face pressure to submit to corporate takeover. The many issues that generated resistance to the corporate option at UCIMC have remained relevant throughout the country, especially at state-supported teaching hospitals.

## THE IMPACT OF LOCAL ADVOCACY

Local advocacy concerning indigent health care in this county led to modest improvements in programs. Increased access, less restrictive eligibility determination, and additional funding for prenatal care and community clinics expanded available services. Without the work of health advocates, proposed cuts in local services would surely have been deeper and more devastating. Advocacy was effective to the extent that a countywide coalition was able to coordinate several strategies: generating meaningful data, developing a politically active coalition of community advocates, and pursuing legal options. Moreover, this advocacy contributed to the efforts of the coalition that successfully resisted corporate takeover of the public teaching hospital that provided disproportionate services to poor people throughout the county.

Each of these strategies has revealed both strengths and weaknesses. Research to document local barriers to care attracted wide attention in a specific area and affected policy decisions, yet such research involved technical compromises that limited its generalizability or pertinence in other localities. Political activism that targeted the policies of county government and local health care institutions succeeded in improving access to services, but these time-consuming and largely defensive efforts did not lead to more creative or proactive programs. Although legal work assisted specific clients in obtaining needed care, the litigation required to improve services for larger groups of patients, such as the undocumented, became difficult to pursue.

While certain circumstances in this county were unique, these experiences may prove helpful to groups advocating for the medically indigent in other localities. Organized advocacy efforts take place frequently in many parts of the United States, although such work does not attract wide attention. Despite variability in local conditions, medical advocacy gains strength from a multifaceted strategy, tailored to local needs, political climate, and existing policies. In developing such a strategy, activists generally can enhance their impact if they include components of short-term research, political work aiming to reduce barriers to access, and focused legal action based on cases whose resolution can lead to policy change.

On the other hand, the piecemeal approach that local health advocates must take does not produce a well organized health care system. Based on such efforts, it is clear that only a national health program that ensures universal entitlement to needed services will lead to the desired outcome: a just and accessible system for all U.S. residents. While we work toward this long-term goal, health advocates can only continue to hold the line in seeking programmatic and funding improvements for the medically indigent in local communities. Sharing information about successful and unsuccessful strategies can enhance such advocacy efforts on the local level.

## ACKNOWLEDGMENT

I gratefully acknowledge the important contributions of Vicki Mayster, Chauncey Alexander, Jean Forbath, Nancy Rimsha, Barbara Akin, Luis de la Maza, Susan Eastman, Carole Harris, F. Allan Hubbell, James Meeker, Hooshang Meshkinpour, Ivette Peña, Nieves Rubio, Lloyd Rucker, Jerome Tobis, and Scott Wylie to the work described in this chapter.

# ◆ chapter seven ◆

# A National Health Program for the United States

B ECAUSE OF THE DEEPENING CRISIS created by the problems of access and costs, both locally and nationally, a national health program for the United States has cycled on and off the policy agenda for many years. Unsuccessful proposals for such a program span three-quarters of a century of U.S. history, so the pace of passage and implementation remains in doubt. During the first years of the Clinton administration, another cycle of intense debate occurred, but proposals again suffered defeat. As a result, the United States remains the only economically developed country without a national health program that provides universal entitlement to health care services.[1] Yet since the underlying problems of access and costs have persisted and actually have continued to worsen in many respects, the need for a national health program still remains recognized by broad segments of the U.S. population.[2]

Although policy debates change quickly and often focus on much more limited reforms, two options have remained as the most prominent proposals for a national program: Those based on managed care versus those based on a single-payer system modeled broadly along the lines of Canada's national health program. At the outset, I should make it clear that I helped

153

develop the single-payer proposal and that the following discussion favors the single-payer approach.[3] While I take a more critical view of managed care as an organizing principle for a U.S. national health program, the references include defenses of this approach that can be reviewed to obtain more information about proponents' views.

## HISTORY OF PRIOR PROPOSALS

Although advocacy for a national health program dates back to the mid-1920s, with the proposal of the Committee on the Costs of Medical Care,[4] the most intense efforts occurred during the 1970s, when the U.S. Congress considered at least 18 separate proposals. The supporters of these measures ranged across a wide political spectrum, including the Nixon administration, the American Medical Association, and both liberal and conservative legislators. During the Reagan and Bush administrations from 1981 to 1992, however, a policy of cutbacks in health and welfare programs eliminated the possibility of enactment. A national health program again emerged as a priority during the 1992 presidential campaign.

Within the range of national health program proposals considered during the late 1970s, several problems became clear. First, the national health program would have changed payment mechanisms, rather than the organization of the health care system. Under these proposals, the federal government would have guaranteed payment for most health services. However, the national health program would not have ensured that practitioners would work in different ways, in different areas, or with different patients.

Most of these plans for the national health program would not have covered all needed medical services. Co-insurance provisions would have required out-of-pocket payment for some fixed percentage of health spending. Such co-payments exert a detrimental impact on the poor and other vulnerable groups, for whom such out-of-pocket payments have been found to exert a substantial disincentive to obtaining needed care.[5]

New and compulsory taxation, usually as fixed payroll deductions, would have paid for the national health program.

The financing arrangements therefore would have been regressive; that is, low-income people would have paid a proportionately higher part of their income for health care than would the wealthy. Although various tax mechanisms could relieve the burden of health insurance for low-income patients, legislators devoted little attention to this issue.

In most national health program plans, private insurance companies would have served as the fiscal intermediaries for the national health program. They would have received compensation for distributing national health program payments from the government to health providers. Such provisions thus would have assured continued profits for the private insurance industry and would have done little to reduce the administrative waste that has characterized this industry.

Regarding accessibility, national health program proposals would have contained few provisions for improving geographic maldistribution of health professionals. Fee schedules might have been higher in some proposals for doctors who practiced in underserved areas, but such incentives could not ensure that physicians actually would work in these areas.

## PERSPECTIVES FROM OTHER COUNTRIES

Planning for a national health program in the United States requires open-minded consideration of the strengths and weaknesses of existing national health programs around the world. For instance, most countries in Western Europe and Scandinavia have initiated national health program structures, permitting private practice in addition to a strong public sector. Canada has achieved universal entitlement to health care through a national health program that depends on private practitioners, private hospitals, and strong planning and coordinating roles for the national and provincial governments.[6]

National health programs vary widely in the degree to which the national government employs health professionals and owns health institutions. For example, the national health programs of the United Kingdom, Denmark, and the Netherlands contract with self-employed general practitioners for primary care; Canadian private practitioners receive public insurance payments mainly on a fee-for-service basis; in Finland and Sweden, a high proportion of practicing doctors work as salaried employees of government agencies. In the United Kingdom, the national government owns most hospitals; regional or local governments own many hospitals in Sweden, Finland, and other Scandinavian countries; and Canada's system depends on governmental budgeting for both public and private hospitals.

The Canadian system is very pertinent to the United States, because of geographic proximity and cultural similarity. Canada assures universal entitlement to health services through a combination of national and provincial insurance programs. Doctors generally receive public insurance payments by fee-for-service arrangements. Hospitals obtain public funds through prospectively negotiated contracts, eliminating the need to bill for specific services. Progressive taxation finances the Canadian system, and the private insurance industry does not play a major role in the program's administration. Most Canadian provinces have initiated policies that aim to correct remaining problems of access based on geographic maldistribution. Cost controls in Canada depend on contracted global budgeting with hospitals, limitations on reimbursements to practitioners (this policy remains controversial for physicians in some provinces), and markedly lower administrative expenses because of reduced eligibility, billing, and collection procedures.

Because of the commonly expressed concern about costs in the United States, the experiences of existing national health programs are instructive. U.S. health care expenditures, already the highest in the world, account for approximately 14 percent of the gross domestic product. The presumption that a national health program would increase costs is not necessarily correct; depending on how it is organized, costs might well fall to below their prior level. First of all, a major savings would come from reduced administrative overhead for billing, collection procedures, eligibility determinations, and other bureaucratic functions that no longer would be necessary. In the Canadian national health program, for instance, global budgeting for hospitals has greatly reduced administrative costs, and a much smaller role for the private insurance industry has lowered costs even further by restricting corporate profit. An analysis by the U.S. General Accounting Office showed that due to savings from reduced administrative functions and entrepreneurialism, a single-payer national health program such as Canada's, if introduced in the United States, would lead to negligible added costs despite achieving universal access to care.[7]

PRINCIPLES AND PROSPECTS FOR
A U.S. NATIONAL HEALTH PROGRAM

National health program proposals can be appraised against several basic principles:[8]

- The national health program would provide for comprehensive care, including diagnostic, therapeutic, preventive, rehabilitative, environmental, and occupational health services, dental and eye care, transportation to medical facilities, social work, and counseling.

- These services generally would not require out-of-pocket payments at the "point of delivery." While carefully limited co-payments for certain services may be appropriate (as in Canada), the implementation of co-payments would ensure that they do not become barriers to access.

- Coverage would be portable, so that travel or relocation has no effect on a person's ability to obtain health care.

- Financing for the national health program would come from a variety of sources, including continued corporate taxation, "healthy taxes" on cigarettes and alcoholic beverages, "conservation taxes" on fossil fuels and other energy sources, "pollution taxes" on known sources of air and water pollution, and a restructured individual tax. Taxation would be progressive, in that individuals and corporations with higher incomes would pay taxes at a higher rate.

- The national health program would reduce administrative costs, private profit, and wasteful procedures in the health care system. A national commission would establish a generic formulary of approved drugs, devices, equipment, and supplies. A national trust fund would disburse payments to private and public health facilities through global and prospective budgeting. Profit to private insurance companies and other corporations would be closely restricted.

- Professional associations would regionally negotiate the fee structures for health care practitioners. Financial incentives would encourage cost control measures through health maintenance organizations, community health centers, and a plurality of practice settings.

- To improve geographic maldistribution of health professionals, the national health program would subsidize education and training in return for required periods of service by medical graduates in underserved areas.

- The national health program would initiate programs of prevention that emphasize individual responsibility for health, risk reduction (including programs to reduce smoking, alcoholism, and substance abuse), nutrition, maternal and infant care, occupational and environmental health, long-term services for the elderly, and other efforts to promote health.

- Elected community representatives would work with providers' groups in local advisory councils. These councils would participate in quality assurance efforts, planning, and obtaining feedback to encourage responsiveness to local needs.

There is and has been wide support for a national health program in the United States. Public opinion polls have shown that a majority of the U.S. population favors a national policy that ensures universal entitlement to basic health care services. Professional organizations including the American Medical Association, the American College of Physicians, the American Public Health Association, and Physicians for a National Health Program—a major physicians' organization favoring a single-payer option—have called for a national health program. Leaders and members of corporations, senior citizens' groups, and a large number of civic organizations have pressed

Congress to create a national health program, although specific proposals have varied. Likewise, many state legislatures have considered setting up state health programs to provide universal access to care.

Strong opposition to a national health program will continue to come from the corporations that currently benefit from the lack of an appropriate national policy: the private insurance industry, pharmaceutical and medical equipment firms, and the for-profit health care chains. Although corporate resistance should not be underestimated, there is also support for a national health program from the corporate world. The costs of private sector medicine have become a major burden to many nonmedical companies that provide health insurance as a fringe benefit to employees. Corporations that do not directly profit from health care have influenced public policy in the direction of cost containment. In Western Europe and Scandinavia, corporations have come to look kindly on the cost controls and services that national health programs provide, even when corporate taxation contributes to the programs' financing.

## A NATIONAL HEALTH PROGRAM BASED ON MANAGED CARE

Proposals for managed care as the basis of a national health program have been complex and have changed over time. The Clinton administration presented a lengthy proposal that received wide attention during the mid-1990s but ultimately was defeated by a broad coalition of interest groups. Although Clinton did not pursue this proposal in the later years of his presidency, its framework has remained the basis of other proposals, and the managed care approach likely will persist in future proposals. My purpose here is to summarize the key features of managed care as the central principle of a national health program and some of the major concerns that have been raised about this approach.

Managed care, although difficult to define simply since it encompasses diverse organizational structures, generally refers to administrative control over the organization and practice of health services, through large corporate entities. Historically, managed care has included such prepaid approaches as health maintenance organizations (HMOs), preferred-provider organizations (PPOs), and proposals for national programs organized by principles of administrative control and market competition. Managed care assumes that quality of care is assured through administrative control and through competition in the marketplace.

The first proposals for a national health program based on managed care appeared during the 1970s. In 1977, Alain Enthoven, an economist whose prior career had focused on military policy analysis at the U.S. Department of Defense and corporations serving as military contractors, offered to the Carter administration a proposal for a "Consumer Choice Health Plan," based on "regulated competition in the private sector." This proposal built in part on prior initiatives by Paul Ellwood for a national "health maintenance strategy" and by Scott Fleming for "structured competition within the private sector."[9] Although Carter rejected the plan, Enthoven soon afterward published the proposal in the medical literature[10] and in a separate monograph.[11] This plan, which presented the basic conceptual structure of all subsequent proposals for national health programs based on managed care, contained important concepts from the military policy work that Enthoven had spearheaded a few years earlier at the Pentagon.[12]

During the 1980s, Enthoven collaborated with Ellwood, other proponents of HMOs, corporate executives, and officers of private insurance companies in developing refinements to the proposal. An emphasis on "managed competition" arose during the mid-1980s in response to concerns raised by economists and business leaders that the original proposal conveyed free market assumptions requiring modification through closer "management" of the program.[13] After publication of a revised proposal in 1989,[14] the coalition supporting managed competition broadened to include officials of the largest U.S. private insurance companies that were diversifying into managed care. These business leaders entered into continuing meetings with Enthoven and other proponents of managed competition at Ellwood's Wyoming home, as part of the so-called "Jackson

Hole group." The managed care sector of the private insurance industry provided major funding for the Jackson Hole group, as well as financial and logistic support for the Clinton presidential campaign and consultation for the Presidential Health Care Task Force.[15]

Although most proposals for managed competition have emerged from this intellectual tradition,[16] certain proposals have suggested modifications in the conceptual structure outlined by Enthoven and colleagues. For instance, although managed competition traditionally has encouraged employer-sponsored plans with participation by private insurance companies, other proposals have separated employment from insurance through the creation of a single, tax-financed, globally budgeted public fund, which would contract with private plans for a minimum benefit package.[17] All managed competition proposals, however, incorporate concepts initiated by Enthoven and colleagues, and all of them call for large-scale changes in the ways medicine is practiced and choices are made by physicians and consumers.

There are four essential features of managed competition. The first element involves large organizations of health care providers. As described in the Clinton proposal, these "accountable health partnerships" (AHPs) are large, integrated organizations of insurers and providers that would offer health plans competitively. Large businesses would participate in these partnerships. The AHPs would operate much as do current managed care organizations (MCOs) and would drastically reduce medical practice based on fee-for-service reimbursement. Instead, physicians and hospitals would be largely absorbed into MCOs. In principle, this shift in the organization of medical practice would allow more stringent management of practice conditions by high-level managers, whose responsibility would be to control costly and self-interested actions by physicians and hospitals.

A second major element of the proposal involves large organizations of purchasers. The Clinton proposal referred to these organizations as "health insurance purchasing cooperatives" (HIPCs); similar proposals have used somewhat different names. Such organizational purchasers would buy health plans from the large organizations of health care providers (AHPs in the Clinton plan). Organized mainly by state governments, these large purchasers would represent small employers and individuals, including both self-employed and unemployed people. In theory, these large "intelligent purchasers" would make informed decisions about costs and quality of services. Under managed competition, Medicaid and possibly Medicare eventually would be privatized and converted to sponsorship by state-organized purchasers.

A uniform benefits package, referred to as "uniform effective health benefits" (UEHB) in the Clinton proposal, is the third essential component of a national health program based on managed care. This benefits package would be extended to the entire population. An appointed national health board would define the minimum benefits contained in the package. This board's decisions about coverage would rely mainly on research about the outcomes and effectiveness of health services.

Tax code changes constitute the fourth essential element of a national health program based on managed care. These changes would restrict the ability of corporations and individuals to claim tax deductions for health care expenditures. Specifically, corporations and individuals could not claim tax deductions for coverage that exceeds the basic coverage provided by the uniform benefits package. Although corporations and individuals could buy additional coverage without tax deductions, these changes in tax code would provide incentives to purchase less expensive coverage overall.

Advocates of a managed care approach to a national health program claim several advantages of this approach. First, it would expand access to health services while still preserving a major role for the private insurance industry. Insurance companies, for instance, could run large managed care programs as fundamental parts of AHPs. As a result, this approach would create less drastic changes in the U.S. health system than a single-payer plan and thus, proponents argue, would stand a better chance of passage in Congress. Because managed care would rely on market forces for cost containment, according to advocates, it would prove more consistent with mainstream political and economic values. Competition, from this view, would lead to improved quality, since managed care plans would have to compete with one another for patients. In selecting among competitive plans, consumers also would need to become more informed about cost-effective care, partly because they would be required to pay co-payments for most services.

Several unknowns have persisted in proposals for managed competition, and the congressional debate on the Clinton administration proposal was unable to clarify these issues fully as managed competition was considered. The extent of the basic benefits to be covered under a national program remained to be worked out. Details of how a national program based on managed competition would be financed, in particular the tax increases to be borne by families and corporations, were not clearly specified. This question about the specifics of projected tax code changes was important, since estimates of the additional costs of a national health program based on managed competition ranged from $30 billion to $100 billion per year. Whether overall health care expenditures would be capped through a global budgeting mechanism remained ambiguous. How transition would occur from the present system to managed competition was not clarified. Further, the degree to which state governments would enjoy flexibility to enact varying forms of coverage and organization remained under debate.

Both supporters and opponents have raised major concerns about managed care as the basis of a national health program.[18] Demographic limitations would restrict its impact, since about 30 percent of the U.S. population lives outside metropolitan areas that could support three or more competing managed care plans. Proponents of managed care have emphasized these demographic limitations to the success of a national health program based on managed care principles. Whether managed care could control costs remains unclear; states with the most extensive managed care programs have shown costs as high as or higher than elsewhere. Administrative costs, already more than 25 percent of overall health care expenditures, likely would increase still further, since managed care is administratively intensive and new organizational sponsors would introduce additional managerial layers.[19] Despite an intent to use research on effectiveness and outcomes to define the uniform minimum benefits package and to assess quality of care, such research has produced verified data about only a small number of medical conditions and procedures.

Several practical questions also have arisen concerning acceptability of a national health program based on managed care to providers and consumers.[20] While expanding the decision-making power of large insurance companies, a national health program based on managed care probably would reduce consumers' freedom to choose practitioners, and micromanagement of clinical decisions likely would increase. Because the ability to buy additional coverage beyond the basic benefits package would depend on income, this provision would perpetuate unequal, multitiered coverage. Whether a national program would succeed in curbing insurance companies' selection or exclusion of patients by risk of costly illness remains in doubt. Managed care likely would create higher out-of-pocket payments and taxes for a substantial part of the population who currently are insured. Furthermore, several polls have shown less public support for managed care as the basis of a national health program than for other alternatives.[21] Evidence that managed care would solve the access problem, while controlling costs remains uncertain.[22] Importantly, it is not clear whether a national health program could successfully address the problems and tensions that managed care has introduced into the patient–doctor relationship, as discussed in chapter 4.

The powerful coalition built up around managed care as the basis for a national program did not succeed in enacting this policy. Although it addressed some of the concerns raised about managed competition, the Clinton team did not agree to change the basic structure of the proposal. This reluctance to consider other options seriously may have stemmed partly from the support that the Clinton campaign received from the managed care sector of the private insurance industry,[23] as well as a perception that simpler and more popular options, including a single-payer approach, were unlikely to pass Congress.

Failure to achieve a workable national health program generated great disappointment, as well as financial waste. Some analysts have believed that the failure of managed care was a necessary step toward the adoption of a simpler approach such as a single-payer option. A less sanguine view holds that the Clinton failure has led to retrenchment, cutbacks, and reinforcement for the paradox of pervasive access barriers coupled with high costs.

Ultimately, as the claims of managed care have become more doubtful in their historical context, should market principles of competition be accepted as cornerstones of national health policy? At the time that he was pursuing military policy at the Pentagon, Enthoven—who has remained the chief intellectual force behind managed care—equated the art of weapon systems analysis and the art of medicine: "Beyond its uniqueness and eclecticism, I would like to say that the art of weapon systems analysis, like the art of medicine, should be based on scientific method, using that term in its broadest sense."[24]

As I have written elsewhere, the conceptual framework of managed competition emerged directly from theories and methods developed initially for military policies that ultimately proved unsuccessful.[25] An alternative vision might be that enunciated by Wendell Berry, a noted farmer and social critic:

> Rats and roaches live by competition under the law of supply and demand; it is the privilege of human beings to live under the laws of justice and mercy. It is impossible not to notice how little the proponents of the ideal of competition have to say about honesty, which is the fundamental economic virtue, and how *very* little they have to say about community, compassion, and mutual help.[26]

## A SINGLE-PAYER NATIONAL HEALTH PROGRAM

This option would provide universal entitlement to needed health care while controlling costs through a single-payer financing system. A single-payer, or "monopsony," financial structure has achieved substantial savings by reducing administrative waste in the national health programs of Canada, Sweden, and Australia. Although none of these programs is without problems, all have minimized barriers to access while controlling costs.

The following features of a single-payer option are based on the proposals of Physicians for a National Health Program (PNHP), of which I am a founding member. The summary provided here leaves out details that are given in national publications to which many colleagues and I have contributed.[27] From its initiation in 1985, PNHP has grown as a national organization to include more than 7,000 members, who are physicians and other health professionals spanning all specialties, states, age groups, and practice settings. Participants in PNHP have come together with a common perception that the problems of access and costs are intolerable, and a belief that a single-payer national health program will remove barriers to access while controlling costs. Although supported by a substantial proportion of the U.S. population in polls, a single-payer system was not the option proposed by the Clinton administration. (Administration leaders privately expressed the view that the single-payer approach was simpler and potentially more effective but acknowledged the political and financial support that the private insurance industry was providing for the managed care approach.)[28] On the other hand, a single-payer approach did emerge as one of the two options for a national health program under consideration in the U.S. Congress.

Coverage under the single-payer proposal would be universal; everyone would be covered. The national health program would provide comprehensive coverage for all medically necessary care, including long-term care. Under this plan, there would be no out-of-pocket costs or co-payments for needed services. Co-payments are not preferred, since they have been found to be substantial disincentives to needed care among low-income patients. Further, co-payments would not be necessary, because costs would be controlled by a single, publicly financed plan that would greatly curtail administrative waste and would achieve cost reductions through monopsony financing. A single-payer national health program would eliminate competing private insurance. This approach would facilitate cost control and discourage multiple tiers of care for different

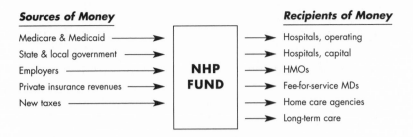

**FIGURE 7.1** *Financial structure of a single-payer national health program.*

income groups, but of course would engender opposition from the wealthy and powerful private insurance industry.

Under a single-payer national health program, hospitals would receive payment through a global budgeting system. The very costly billing apparatus, which is responsible for unnecessary administrative costs in hospitals under the present system, would be eliminated. Instead, hospitals would negotiate an annual global budget for all operating costs. It is important to note that hospitals would remain privately owned and run, rather than becoming part of a nationalized ownership structure. To reduce overlapping and duplicative facilities that increase overall costs, capital purchases and expansion would be budgeted separately, based on regional health planning goals. Regional health planning boards, with members elected by consumers and providers, would make these decisions about capital expenditures and expansion.

The national health program would collect and disburse virtually all payments for health services (figure 7.1). This single-payer structure would provide the major overall source of cost control. Total expenditures would be capped at the proportion of the gross domestic product spent for health services during the year prior to implementation of the national health program. Initially, during a transition period of approximately three years, funding would come from existing sources to minimize economic disruption: Medicare and Medicaid, state and local governments, employers, and private insurance premiums. After the transition period, the collection of payments would be converted to a simplified process based on taxation, in which the average company, individual, and family would pay approximately the same in taxes as was previously paid in insurance premiums, deductibles, co-payments, and other out-of-pocket spending. (A PNHP publication provides further details about these financing mechanisms.)[29] The national health program would distribute payments for services to hospitals, MCOs, physicians, home care agencies, and long term care agencies.

Payment for physicians and ambulatory care would occur under one of three options. First, physicians could choose to be paid on a fee-for-service basis. Under this option, state medical associations would negotiate a simplified fee schedule for the range of covered services; practitioners would accept fees as payment in full and would not bill patients separately, except for a small number of uncovered services, such as purely cosmetic surgery. As a second option, the national health program would provide capitation payments to MCOs employing salaried physicians. However, provisions of this option would protect against possible abuses seen under prior managed care programs; for instance, free disenrollment privileges would be required, and MCOs would be prohibited from selective enrollment of healthier patients. Capitation fees would cover operating costs only, rather than capital purchases, profits, or physician incentives. Under the capitation option, global budgeting would apply to inpatient care. The third option for physician payment would involve salaries received from globally budgeted institutions, such as hospitals, community clinics, and home care agencies.

The national health program would cover all needed drugs and medical supplies. An expert board would develop a national formulary based on principles of generic drug substitution and assurance of high standards of biological quality. As far as possible, reimbursement procedures would encourage the use of less expensive generic alternatives. This provision would reduce the excessive costs incurred from the promotion and detailing of new drugs without greater demonstrated efficacy than less expensive formulations.

How would the national health program look from the patient's point of view? First, universal access to comprehensive care would remove barriers to access. There would be no out-of-pocket costs, and patients would have free choice of doctors and hospitals. Hassles in using and processing private or public insurance would be reduced through the implementation of a single program for everyone.

From the practitioner's point of view, conditions of practice would improve considerably, especially because the wallet biopsy—that emotionally and ethically degrading procedure that physicians often must use before deciding how to diagnose or treat a patient—no longer would be necessary. Instead, the national health program would fully cover all needed services. Doctors would most likely experience greater clinical freedom and less intrusive micromanagement by administrators. In addition, physicians would be free to choose from a variety of practice settings. Overall, there would be little change in anticipated income; as in Canada, practitioners in the primary care specialties could anticipate equal or somewhat greater earnings than previously, and only the highest paid surgical subspecialists could expect to see a fall in income.

From the corporate viewpoint, companies would experience a stabilization in costs of health care. Those corporations that currently provide health insurance as a fringe benefit of employment likely would see a reduction in health care expenses; projections for automobile manufacturers such as Ford or Chrysler indicate that costs would decline more than $4,000 per employee per year. Companies that do not currently provide health insurance as a fringe benefit would experience higher costs, but the single-payer national health program would provide subsidies for small businesses that are at greatest financial risk. The economic competitiveness of U.S. corporations overall would increase, as companies would incur health care costs more in line with those of their international competitors.

In summary, a single-payer national health program would provide universal, comprehensive coverage, without out-of-pocket payments. Hospitals would be paid a global, lump-sum operating budget, to be negotiated annually. Capital budgets for hospitals would be negotiated based on regional health planning goals. Physicians and ambulatory care would be paid through one of three options: fee-for-service, capitation in HMOs, or salary in globally budgeted institutions. A single public payer would control costs and achieve public accountability while minimizing administrative waste. Simplicity and international experience with the single-payer approach make it a reasonable alternative for a U.S. national health system, but rationality by no means guarantees political success.

## CONCLUSION

The political process surrounding a national health program, as practiced in the United States, conveys an overall sense of irrationality and lack of coherent policy. This irrationality and incoherence become even more apparent from an overview of the comparative costs of various local and national policies. For instance, initiating a single-payer national health program that would solve the access problem while controlling costs would incur very little additional expense, certainly on an order of magnitude less than current expenditures on possibly outdated or unnecessary military systems, such as the Stealth bomber, as well as public support of the private financial sector in such efforts as the savings-and-loan bailout. On the other hand, as estimated by the U.S. Congressional Budget Office, a national health program based on managed care would represent a substantial increase in expenditures, on the order of $80 billion per year.[30]

For better or worse, the lack of a national health program will continue to plague the United States. The chronic crisis of U.S. health policy gives reasons for pessimism, but also clarifies some of the opportunities that await us in trying to construct more humane society and health care system.

# ◆ chapter eight ◆

# Needed Changes in Society

WHILE A NATIONAL HEALTH PROGRAM would address the terrible problems of access and costs in the United States, it would not correct other problems that are rooted in the structure of U.S. society. But to clarify: The United States urgently needs a national health program that provides universal access to services. Until this goal is accomplished, this richest and most powerful country in the world will continue to distinguish itself as the only economically developed country that does not assure access through a coherent national policy. This uncivilized situation paradoxically coincides with the highest expenditures on health care per capita among all nations. In short, the achievement of a successful national health program must remain our most important objective, despite opposition that comes from economically powerful interest groups.

On the other hand, we should not delude ourselves by expecting that the achievement of a national health program in the United States will attain urgently needed improvements in health outcomes. In this country, mortality and other health outcomes are closely linked to patterns of inequality based on class, race, and gender. Some data on life expectancy and outcomes for specific diseases (recapped from chapter 3) clarify these associations, which are unlikely to be corrected by policy changes affecting health care alone.

## SOCIAL DIFFERENTIALS IN MORTALITY
## AND HEALTH OUTCOMES

Although U.S. death rates declined somewhat since 1960, low-income and poorly educated people still die at higher rates than those with greater income or better education.[1] Multiple studies have continued to show much higher mortality rates among the poor, not only overall, but also for a large number of specific disease processes. For instance, this research has found worse outcomes for cancer, cardiovascular disease, and arthritic conditions among low-income people. Most cardiovascular risk factors, such as hypertension, obesity, physical inactivity, and diabetes mellitus, occur with a higher prevalence among people with lower socioeconomic status. On the other hand, unhealthy behaviors among poor people explain relatively little variance in adverse health outcomes, as compared with lower socioeconomic status itself.[2] In short, social class—especially related to low income—remains a very powerful predictor of illness and early death.

Regarding the impact of race and gender, African Americans and Native Americans manifest much worse health outcomes and mortality than whites. For instance, as of the mid-1990s, survival until age 65 of African-American males in Harlem was worse than for males in Bangladesh. Average life expectancy in McKinley County, New Mexico, where Native Americans constitute 72 percent of the population, was 72.3 years, compared with the national rate of 75.4. Adverse conditions seemed to affect minority males to a greater extent than females.[3] In addition to overall mortality, African Americans have continued to show much worse outcomes for specific diseases such as cancer, stroke, and kidney failure, as well as maternal mortality. These differences can be partially attributed to access barriers, but they hold even for African Americans who have insurance and apparently adequate access to needed services.[4] Native Americans have experienced an epidemic of adverse outcomes from several diseases, but most dramatically, diabetes mellitus.[5]

In short, several social conditions remain strong determinants of death and disease outcomes in the United States. Poverty and income inequality, which are fundamental features of social class, exert a profound impact on mortality and disease. Among the determinants of health outcomes, social class remains the strongest.[6] Race is the other major social determinant; there is convincing evidence that racism continues to affect health outcomes and the processes of health care, including diagnostic decisions by physicians that affect African Americans adversely in comparison with whites.[7] Gender also affects outcomes, especially for older women, who experience gender bias in diagnostic decision making and who manifest worst outcomes than men of similar social class in such conditions as heart disease, despite the more favorable mortality overall for women.[8]

Within countries that have implemented largely successful national health programs, mortality and other health outcomes have remained linked to social class, despite improvements in access to health care services. Evidence from Canada, the United Kingdom, and Scandinavia has shown that major social differentials in health outcomes, and in access to services, persist even in the context of highly regarded national health programs whose goal is to achieve universal access. For instance, outcomes from several chronic conditions are worse in Canadian provinces with rural and largely Native American populations. Financial barriers to obtaining prescribed medications apparently lead to reduced access and utilization of services by some low-income Canadians.[9]

The important Whitehall study in the United Kingdom found a clear social class gradient of mortality and adverse health outcomes. During the 1980s, research subjects who worked as civil servants with low income and subordinate job positions showed much worse overall mortality and outcomes in specific diseases than workers with higher income and supervisorial job positions. This social class gradient presented itself in the United Kingdom about 40 years after the implementation of the British National Health Service.[10]

In Scandinavia, whose countries manifest more homogeneity in their populations than the United States and have longstanding national programs that assure access to health care services, similar social differentials have emerged. Even when other class-based inequalities are reduced, characteristics of the work process such as time pressure and hierarchical power relationships predict negative health outcomes. In Sweden, which also manifests more homogeneity in its population and has a long-standing national health program, Karasek and Theorell have conducted research about the impact of work on health. They have found that workers who experienced high levels of "strain" in their jobs—which involved increased psychological demand coupled with a lack of decision latitude permitted by supervisors—manifested worse health outcomes than workers who experienced lower levels of strain. This finding has emerged from several studies in Sweden and more recently has been replicated in the United States. Karasek, Theorell, and colleagues have advocated major modifications in workplace relationships as a strategy with positive potential to improve health outcomes through social change.[11]

Solutions to health problems rooted in social class, work hierarchies, race, and gender must flow from wider changes in social policy. Despite the advantages of national policies that provide universal access to health care services, policies restricted to the health sector will not resolve the more fundamental social problems that lie beneath social differentials in mortality and health outcomes, even in countries with national health programs. This conclusion implies the need for social changes that go far beyond the health sector.

Here it is worth considering seriously Salvador Allende's agenda for social policy, as outlined in chapter 3.[12] To recall: During 1939, as minister of health in a progressive Chilean government, Allende and his colleagues studied the major health problems that confronted the nation. Based on epidemiological research concerning infectious diseases, occupational illnesses, obstetrical and perinatal outcomes, alcoholism, malnutrition, and other important problems, Allende concluded that broad social changes would accomplish more to improve the health of the Chilean people than would narrower public health programs or initiatives for improving access to health care services. Instead of public health initiatives per se, Allende called for and began to implement policies of income redistribution, a national housing program, food distribution, reforms in the work process, and environmental protection.

Far from a utopian vision, proposals such as Allende's remain the only directions of change that will address the inequalities of mortality and health outcomes that persist after implementation of a national health program. Even if we succeed in finally establishing a long-overdue national program in the United States, many of the most important social differentials in mortality and health outcomes will remain. Policies must address the root causes of these social differentials, and these root causes remain closely linked to social class, racism, gender inequalities, work hierarchies and exposures, and environmental problems. To achieve fundamental change in these arenas, activism aiming at more fundamental modifications of economic and power relationships must take place. Such activism requires a vision of health praxis that goes beyond the health sector to deal with the root causes of health problems in the broader society.

## HEALTH PRAXIS

*Praxis* is the uniting of theory and practice, study and action.[13] As I have argued, understanding the problems of medicine and society is not enough; knowledge alone will not solve the difficulties that beset us. Research and analysis must be linked to political action. For meaningful improvements in health outcomes, it is important to understand the roots of illness and suffering that extend beyond the health sector, but it is also necessary to move beyond study to the practicalities of change. Therefore, I would like to suggest some directions of progressive health praxis.

Health workers and activists concerned about the relationship between social change and health outcomes face difficult challenges in their day-to-day work. Clients' problems often have roots in the social system. Examples abound: drug addicts and alcoholics who prefer numbness to the pain of unemployment and inadequate housing; persons with occupational diseases that require treatment but will worsen upon return to illness-generating work conditions; housewives harassed by responsibilities at home and lacking opportunities for fulfilling work experience; people with stress-related cardiovascular disease; elderly or disabled people who need periodic medical certification to obtain welfare benefits that are barely adequate; prisoners who develop illnesses because of prison conditions; homeless people whose infectious diseases and mental health problems are inseparable from homelessness itself. Health workers usually feel obliged to respond to the expressed needs of these and many similar clients.

In doing so, however, health workers engage in "patching." On the individual level, patching permits clients' continued functioning in a social system that is often the source of the problem. Patching also involves the sometimes unwitting communication of messages that exert social control and reinforce society's dominant ideologies. At the societal level, the cumulative effect of these interchanges is the patching of a social system whose patterns of oppression frequently cause disease and personal unhappiness.

The medical model that teaches practitioners to serve individual patients deflects attention from this difficult and frightening dilemma. Even health workers who are highly critical of our society devote much of their clinical work to patching the system's victims; frequently this work has the paradoxical effect of preserving the system's overall stability. These observations do not impugn the efforts of caring health workers, but point out some of the unintended consequences of clinical work.

The contradictions of patching have no simple resolution. Clearly, health workers cannot deny services to clients, even when these services permit clients' participation in illness-generating social structures and do not attack the deeper roots of their problems. On the other hand, it is important to draw this connection between social issues and personal troubles.[14] Although the contradictions of patching are difficult for practitioners who want progressive social change, their recognition leads to certain conclusions about health praxis. The most basic conclusion is that health work in itself is not sufficient. Instead, health workers should try to link their clinical activities to efforts aimed directly at basic sociopolitical change. Political action focusing on health care should accompany activism that extends beyond the health care system alone. The goal here is to encourage health praxis that points to progressive change in the social order.

Linking problems of health care to underlying social contradictions must address the social roots of medical problems, and it is important to acknowledge the contradictions of reform. If those working toward health care reforms do not do so, solutions will remain limited and ultimately unsatisfactory. Improved material circumstances may seem beneficial, but ultimately may reinforce the status quo by reducing the potential for social conflict. When oppressive conditions exist, improvements seem reasonable. However, the history of health and welfare reform has shown that reforms most often follow social protest, make incremental improvements that do not change overall patterns of oppression, and face cutbacks when protest recedes.[15]

A distinction developed initially by Gorz clarifies this problem.[16] "Reformist reforms" provide small material improvements while leaving intact current political and economic structures. These reforms may reduce discontent for periods of time, while helping to preserve the system in its present form:

> A reformist reform is one which subordinates objectives to the criteria of rationality and practicability of a given system and policy. . . . [It] rejects those objectives and demands—however deep the need for them—which are incompatible with the preservation of the system.

"Nonreformist reforms" achieve lasting changes in the present system's structures of power and finance. They do not simply modify material conditions; instead, they provide the potential for mass political action. Rather than obscuring sources of exploitation by small incremental improvements, nonreformist reforms expose and highlight structural inequities. Such reforms ultimately increase frustration and political tension in a society; they do not seek to reduce these sources of political energy. As Gorz puts it, such reforms "are to be regarded as a means and not an end, as dynamic phases in a progressive struggle, not as stopping places." From this viewpoint, in health care as in other fields, one tries to discern which reform proposals are reformist and which are nonreformist. One also takes an advocacy role, supporting the latter and opposing the former.

The distinction between reformist and nonreformist reforms is seldom easy. Few reform proposals address the underlying social causes of medical problems. It is essential to understand and to criticize piecemeal reformism. It is also necessary to examine carefully the much smaller number of health reforms and progressive directions of health activism that truly challenge broad social contradictions and that heighten the potential for basic social change. Without these links between medicine and social structure, both problems and solutions will continue to float in a haze of confusion and mystification.

Proposals for national health programs also deserve analysis concerning their potential for reformism. Even the single-payer national health program, if unaccompanied by other work aimed at changing the underlying social determinants of illness and early death, runs the risk of obscuring the more fundamental social changes that are needed. The single-payer proposal includes several key elements that directly challenge existing relationships of power and finance in U.S. society. For instance, by unifying the payment mechanism into a single public structure, and prohibiting parallel private insurance coverage for treatments that are covered under the national public system, the single-payer proposal would change dramatically the dominant position of the private insurance industry, which is currently one of the most powerful sectors in the U.S. political–economic system. In addition, by requiring a national formulary of generic medications, the single-payer proposal challenges the power and exploitative tendencies of the pharmaceutical industry. On the other hand, if the single-payer approach is not coupled with activism to change the underlying social determinants of adverse health outcomes, it will become a reform with important but limited consequences.

Because problems of health care derive in large part from problems of society, strategies for change should deal with this linkage. As an overall strategy, activism exposes, highlights, and in some cases exacerbates the social contradictions that are sources of health problems. These efforts also address the structures of oppression that the social organization of medicine both reflects and helps maintain. Social contradictions create points of weakness and vulnerability. In confronting these contradictions, especially during crises, activism can aim toward nonreformist goals and longer-term change in society. If specific issues in health care have social roots, these interrelationships can become a focus of organizing. Health workers can consider the subtle ways that medical services can permit clients' functioning in a social system that is a source of their difficulties. By taking action to change the social origins of medical problems, health workers and other activists can begin to address the limitations of patching.

For those readers interested in political activism, it may be helpful to think about several concrete alternatives for action. The overview that follows is not exhaustive, nor does it provide straightforward solutions to the problems raised here. Concerning the practicalities of political action, there is bound to be disagreement. Directions of activism also predictably will shift over time. The purpose is to convey the range of nonreformist strategies that trace medical problems to underlying conditions of society and then to specify some priorities.

Class structure in the health care system mirrors the more general contradictions of social class. Members of the corporate and upper-middle classes dominate the policy-making bodies of North American health care institutions. But coalitions of community residents and health workers have tried to gain greater control of medical centers, hospitals, and clinics. In communities resisting the expansion of private medical centers, local residents have demanded positions on the boards of these institutions. Through this participation, low-income community members have exerted pressure to limit expansion and obtain needed services.

While private medical centers have expanded, public hospitals have contracted; besides reducing services, public-sector cutbacks have led to layoffs and unemployment for many health workers. Community-worker coalitions have played a key role in resisting cutbacks in services and closures of public hospitals. Community organizing also has led to the formation of locally controlled clinics, whose clients elect representatives to make policy decisions. Workers at these clinics usually participate in policy making. The success of community-worker coalitions has varied in different localities. In many areas, activism by these coalitions has led to more accessible and responsive services, as well as broader participation by community residents and workers in health policy.

Class structure also manifests itself in the stratification of workers within health care institutions. Union organizing, which has occurred in medical centers throughout the United States, can modify this stratification. In the past, different professional orientations have caused technicians, nurses, doctors, and other groups to start separate unions. These groups generally negotiate with the same administrators and governing boards, but often with a reduced power base because of professional divisions. In countering the divisive impact of professionalism, the unionization effort may try to overcome these divisions. Unionization in health care also can go beyond narrow economic goals. Although workers' economic interests are important, unions can seek greater control over the work process and participation in policy making. Union organizing in health care is not an end in itself but can be a useful strategy when it aims toward wider shifts in political and economic power.[17]

Racism heightens the impact of class structure in the health care system. To address the combined effects of racism and social class, minority groups have organized to increase their recruitment into medicine and obtain better medical care. Minority caucuses have formed at many health science schools. Chicano, Puerto Rican, black, and other minority organizations have created programs to improve services in local communities and oppose racism in medicine. Affirmative action to combat racism has achieved only limited success. After increases in the admission of blacks to medical schools in the late 1960s and early 1970s, enrollment subsequently declined again, and recruitment of minorities into the health professions has de-

creased even further due to legal rulings and legislative man-
dates that have weakened the principles of affirmative action.[18]
Similarly, although the utilization of medical services by minorities rose after the passage of Medicaid and Medicare legislation
during the 1960s, problems such as high infant mortality and
adverse outcomes from diseases such as cancer and cardiovascular disorders still disproportionately affect minorities. These
issues will continue to be a focus for activists concerned with
racism in health care.

Despite periods of economic growth, the economy remains
volatile, with frequent and recurrent crises. Uneven development persists, as rural areas and low-income urban districts
face a maldistribution of medical and other needed services.
The private–public contradiction, by which public funds subsidize private medical centers and corporations while public
facilities face cutbacks, worsens such inequities even further.

Attempts to expand private medical centers and achieve
corporate takeover of public medical centers have occurred frequently in the health care system. In many cities, the growth of
private hospitals and medical schools has threatened housing
and the survival of low-income communities. Activists have
organized against private medical expansion. Most often, planning provisions, which are supposed to assess the need for
expansion and control costs, have had very little impact. Organizers in several cities, however, have stopped unnecessary
expansion and corporate takeover. In others, low-income residents have obtained positions on the governing boards of private medical centers.

Organizing against private medical expansion also calls
attention to the many forms of public subsidization of the private sector. These subsidizations include public payment for
low-income patients, government grants and loans for new construction, and tax advantages because of private hospitals' nonprofit status. Such uses of public moneys weaken public-sector
medicine, whose funding tends to decline as private medical
centers expand. Meanwhile, private hospitals still try to transfer
uninsured patients to public facilities; despite federal legislation
restricting this practice, the "dumping" of indigent patients

from the private to the public sector still warrants organizing. Political activism that opposes private expansion and aims toward a stronger public sector is a key part of health praxis.

Other work, based largely in medical schools and hospitals, deals with the profits of large corporations and advocates a reduction of private finance capital in reorganization of the health care system. For example, in researching the financial operations of private medical centers, activists have uncovered major sources of profit for banks, trusts, and insurance companies. Despite their nonprofit status, many private hospitals accept loans and investments from financial institutions that later receive high rates of interest. Frequently, officers of the same financial institutions sit on the governing boards of the hospitals that obtain loans and investments. Local organizers have worked to publicize and change these economic relationships. At the national level, activists also have called for a reduction of private finance capital in medicine. This work, for instance, has opposed the role of the private insurance industry in publicly funded insurance programs, managed care organizations, and peer review.

The "medical-industrial complex," especially the pharmaceutical and medical equipment industries, has drawn heavy criticism for promoting costly, ineffective technology and exploiting illness for private profit. Locally, organizers in hospitals and community clinics have insisted on the development of generic drug formularies and have opposed the promotion of drugs within their institutions by pharmaceutical company representatives. Similar actions by medical and nursing students have prevented the use of misleading educational materials from drug houses.

Another important local effort emphasizes expensive technology at private medical centers. Corporations develop and promote technological innovations such as coronary care units, fetal monitoring systems, and radiologic scanning devices. Although their effectiveness in improving morbidity and mortality is largely unverified, private medical centers buy these devices in an uncoordinated fashion. The proliferation of technology increases the costs of medical care and diverts attention from simpler services that are sorely needed. Organizers in several cities have rallied opposition against private hospitals' purchase of advanced technologies, especially when these institutions do not provide adequate medical care to low-income residents.

Policies of the state continue to protect the economic system based in private profit and monopoly capital. The state supports the private sector, for example, by public subsidization of expanding medical centers and firms doing business in medical products. The state also helps legitimate the current social order by providing health and welfare services in the public sector. Especially during periods of recession, however, the contradictions of state expenditures lead to cutbacks of public services. These cutbacks can have devastating effects on needed medical care. The analysis and redirection of state policies are essential goals for activists concerned about the difficulties that the private–public duality creates.

The impact of medical ideology has motivated attempts to demystify current ideological patterns and develop alternatives. These efforts emphasize the complex etiology of many health problems, the frequent inappropriateness of technological solutions, and the medicalization of social problems. Educational campaigns, often in community clinics or trade unions, focus on illness-generating conditions in the workplace and environment. Several groups have publicized and acted against the growing social control function of medicine in such areas as drug addiction, genetic screening, contraception and sterilization abuse, and psychosurgery. These efforts have heightened sensitivity to the messages of ideology and social control that health professionals transmit within the patient–doctor relationship. The women's and self-help movements have developed less esoteric medical care, which reduces professional dominance and fosters personal autonomy. Alternative health programs also have emerged that try to develop nonhierarchical and noncapitalist forms of practice; these ventures then would be available as models of progressive health work when future political change permits their wider acceptance.[19]

The social contradictions that foster problems of health care extend beyond the national boundaries of the United States. Political activism can address these international issues. One concern is the foreign operation of the pharmaceutical and medical equipment industries. Multinational corporations have cultivated markets abroad for expensive technologies; often these technologies are inappropriate in the context of underdevelopment, when more basic needs cannot be met. Pharmaceutical companies have used people in Third World countries for testing of drugs whose safety is unknown; an example is that of oral contraceptives, which drug companies tested and sold in Latin America before their complications became apparent. Moreover, drug houses frequently sell medications in Third World countries when regulatory agencies disapprove their use in the United States because of risks and complications. The promotion of infant formula instead of breast milk in countries where formulas are dangerous because of unsanitary water supplies is another example of exploitative behavior by pharmaceutical companies. Several groups based in North American hospitals and medical schools have documented these activities of the pharmaceutical and equipment industries. This information has been useful both in the United States and abroad to restrict the dumping through export of products that otherwise could not be sold. North American corporations dealing in drugs and equipment benefit greatly from their activities in underdeveloped countries; these activities can be a target of political work in the United States.

Activism also has focused on the linkages between health care and international financial policies.[20] For instance, the policies of the World Bank, International Monetary Fund, and Inter-American Development Bank have required cutbacks in public-sector services within Third World countries as a condition for new or renegotiated loans. These "structural adjustment" policies have led to great difficulties in maintaining a public safety net that provides curative and preventive services to people who do not have access to care outside the public sector. In many instances, such financial policies have fostered the ability of multinational corporations to export for-profit managed care programs to Third World countries, linked to privatization of public health systems and social security funds. These policies have generated widespread resistance by activists who oppose the globalization of multinational corporations' dominance over economic activities in general and health care in particular. In some countries, this activism has slowed the entry of multinational corporations into health care activities and has generated alternative reforms at the local level.

In several countries with totalitarian governments aided by the United States, health workers have suffered imprisonment and torture. Medical professionals supporting dictatorships, on the other hand, have taken part in torture and related activities that have jeopardized their colleagues' safety. Several international groups have formed to assist persecuted health workers and speak out against medical complicity in torture. Publicizing detrimental effects on health and safety, these groups have called for an end to military and economic assistance for such regimes.

Another phase of international work involves support for countries that have undergone progressive change linking medicine and society. Health workers from the United States have traveled to such countries as Cuba, Vietnam, Tanzania, Mozambique, Angola, Zimbabwe, and Nicaragua. These visits, sometimes involving extended stays, generally have served two purposes. In the first place, health workers can provide direct services. Especially during the early years after a revolution, when professionals tend to leave a country because of their threatened class position, visiting health workers can fill a critical need. Second, visitors on their return can spread information about the impact of U.S. foreign policy and about health care in postrevolutionary societies. Health brigades organized in the United States and Western Europe have sent money and medical supplies to countries with severe shortages. The educational work that accompanies these actions fosters further organizing within dominant nations that have been responsible for many damaging effects of imperialism and underdevelopment.

Illness-generating social conditions have important implications for political action. Proof that some occupations are associated with specific disease and mortality patterns has led to interventions in workplaces and unions. Organizations of medical and science workers have taken part in occupational safety and health projects. The purposes of these efforts are to publicize the problems, inform unions and local communities about hazards and possible solutions, and exert pressure on companies and government regulatory agencies for stricter enforcement.

Activists in unions and the women's movement have focused on work- and stress-related illness. They also have recognized the illness-generating potential of economic cycles; this finding has formed one basis of requests for cost-of-living clauses in contracts and job security provisions that would dampen the effects of these cycles. Organizing against sexism has included demands for improved work conditions that recognize differential risks for men and women but rectify discriminatory wage patterns.

Such efforts in occupational and environmental health seek to enhance workers' control over the conditions of work and communities' ability to eliminate environmental hazards. Confronting the contradiction between profit and safety is necessary to modify the social origins of illness. This problem becomes ever more critical, as illness-generating conditions of the workplace and environment threaten humanity's survival.

What are the priorities? The range of nonreformist activism shows many areas in which change is needed; several problems are particularly urgent. Strategies to address these problems deserve high priority.

First, the recurrent fiscal crises of advanced capitalist economies present both dangers and opportunities. Stagnation and cutbacks in health care and other public services heighten tensions throughout the society. The ultra-right has emerged as a well-financed and politically powerful interest group. Some elements of the ultra-right have developed a striking public presence and leadership style. Such organizations reveal an authoritarian fervor that, as many observers have noted, is reminiscent of fascism. At the same time, openly racist groups have grown in size and public visibility; under conditions of economic and political instability, polarization along class and racial lines is likely to deepen. Antiracist activism has become a crucial priority in workplace and community organizing. In the health care system, as community-worker coalitions, unions, and similar organizations go about their work, they should view racism and class as interrelated structures of oppression.

International work, especially in opposition to economic exploitation, is a second priority. Medicine, capitalism, and economic imperialism historically have been intertwined. Medical and public health professionals have played an important and often unwitting role in the exploitation of Third World countries. Dominant nations frequently have tried to maintain their power through direct military intervention, as in Indochina. At other times these efforts are subtler, as in the economic destabilization of new governments or covert military support for dictatorships. The policies of international lending agencies such as the World Bank have led to widespread difficulties as public-sector institutions, which historically have provided a safety net for low-income people, are cut back and privatized. International work will continue as an important focus for progressive action in health care.

Third, there is the inescapable problem of illness-generating conditions in the workplace and environment. During the past two centuries, the world has become a dumping ground for toxic wastes. Environmental exploitation has emerged as a damaging effect of capitalist development, but similar problems also have arisen in socialist countries. Epidemics of cancer and other chronic diseases have appeared among workers in a variety of industries. The hazards of nuclear power and stockpiled weapons threaten humanity and other life forms because of potential accidents as much as the intentional use of these technologies. In capitalist societies, the structure of private profit impedes efforts to deal systematically with occupational and environmental health problems; these medical consequences emerge from the very fabric of our society as currently organized. Changing such social roots of illness-generating conditions has become an essential goal if we are to have a future at all.[21]

Some useful directions of political strategy are clear. Social contradictions lie beneath many medical problems; the social organization of medicine both reflects and fosters structures of oppression. These contradictions and oppressive structures are important targets of political activism. The urgency of such problems justifies impatience, but patience is needed. Because of the resistance it will encounter, the struggle for change will be a protracted one and will involve action on many fronts. The present holds little room for complacency or misguided optimism. Our future health care system, as well as the social order of which it will be a part, depends largely on the praxis we choose now.

## ✦ chapter nine ✦

# Needed Changes in the
# Patient–Doctor Relationship

T HE CHANGES NEEDED AT THE LEVELS of the health care system
and of the society will not come easily. Such transformations require political action that goes beyond the usual limits of
policy proposals. To achieve equitable access to care at reasonable costs, and to achieve improved health outcomes across
social classes and races, fundamental changes in the social structures of our society have to occur. In particular, the social structural issues that stand in the way of a just health care system
need to be confronted, especially the political and economic
power of the private insurance industry; without that confrontation, the United States will retain its distinction as the last
economically developed country without a national health program. Similarly, the societal structures that maintain income and
racial inequalities must change, if meaningful improvements in
health outcomes are to be obtained. These improvements will
not occur even with a successful national health program.

In short, an economically developed country ascribing to
principles of justice must have a national health program that
permits universal access to services. But even more fundamental change in the relationships among social classes and races

must occur to improve the pervasive inequalities in health outcomes that members of our society experience. These themes
have run through the last chapters.

In this final chapter, I want to return to the level of the primary care encounter, recognizing that what goes on in the
encounter, even when aggregated over many encounters, will
have less potential impact on health outcomes than changes
that are needed at much broader levels in our society. Even so,
primary care encounters will continue to occur, both before and
after broader social transformations take place. Improvements
at the "micro" level of the patient–doctor encounter, and how
to get there from here, become a way of concluding this consideration of the quest for solutions.

## DEALING WITH SOCIAL CONTEXT IN
## PATIENT–DOCTOR ENCOUNTERS

Many practitioners feel reluctant to get involved in helping
improve the contextual problems that patients face—no matter
how important such problems may be. Before the growth of
managed care, doctors commonly experienced such reluctance
because they viewed their involvement in patients' contextual
difficulties as beyond the medical role, or because they could
not find the time to extend their role to the contextual arena.
The constraints introduced by managed care have made practitioners' involvement in patients' contextual concerns even
more problematic. For instance, the productivity expectations
and financial structure of managed care discourage efforts to
deal with such problems. Several years ago, members of our
research group on patient–doctor communication and I worked
out some preliminary criteria to guide practitioners in addressing contextual concerns.[1]

These criteria try to address the question: To what extent
*should* physicians intervene in the social context? The answer to
this question depends partly on clarification of the practitioner's role, especially the degree to which intervention in the
social context comes to be seen as appropriate and desirable.
Practitioners reasonably may respond to this analysis by refer-
ring to the time constraints of current practice arrangements,

the need to deal with challenging technical problems, and a lack of support facilities and personnel to improve social conditions. How physicians should involve themselves in contextual difficulties, without increasing professional control in areas where physicians claim no special expertise, therefore takes on a certain complexity.

On the other hand, the presence of social problems in medical encounters warrants more critical attention. Briefly, on the most limited level, physicians should let patients tell their stories with far fewer interruptions, cutoffs, or returns to technical matters. Patients should have the chance to present their narratives in an open-ended way. When patients refer to personal troubles that derive from contextual issues, physicians should try not to marginalize these connections by reverting to a technical track. Although such suggestions encourage more "attentive patient care" and more acknowledgment of patients' contextual stories within medical encounters,[2] some preliminary criteria also may prove helpful for physicians in deciding when and under what circumstances they could initiate, extend, or limit discussions about contextual matters.

First, it is important to recognize that patients differ in their openness and desire for contextual discussion; physicians should take their cues here from the initiative that patients themselves show in raising contextual concerns. For instance, in the encounter with the elderly woman described in chapter 4, the patient introduces extensive contextual material concerning loss of home and community, social isolation, transportation problems, financial insecurity, and nutritional concerns. Rather than supportive listening alone, the physician here might respond more directly to these patient-initiated concerns by mentioning contextual interventions that could prove fairly easy to arrange: referral to seniors' organizations in the patient's new neighborhood, home care services including nursing and nutritional assistance, social work support to help with financial issues, information about transportation services, and efforts to coordinate care with the patient's family members and friends.

Second, under other circumstances, physicians should remain sensitive to patients' differing desires and needs. Some patients may prefer no contextual interventions. Physicians' inquiry about contextual concerns requires tactful recognition of patients' autonomy to limit contextual discussion and to refuse such interventions.

In considering the time and costs devoted to contextual discussion and intervention, a point of concern especially to managed care organizations, a third criterion suggests that physicians and patients consider effects of contextual conditions on outcomes of care, such as prognosis, functional capacity, and satisfaction. Regarding the above encounter, the geriatric literature provides extensive evidence that social isolation, lack of convenient transportation, financial insecurity, and inadequate nutritional support all worsen the functional capacity of older people.[3] Contextual concerns such as isolation and related social psychological problems also can affect morbidity and mortality. Social isolation and psychological distress, for instance, are associated with higher rates of adverse cardiac events after myocardial infarction, and these effects may be equal or greater in magnitude than previously established cardiac risk factors.[4]

Current productivity standards in managed care are leading to tighter scheduling of shorter appointments, which do not encourage the exploration of contextual concerns. When constraints of time and costs require prioritization, existing evidence about the importance of specific contextual problems for health outcomes can help guide physicians and patients in targeting contextual issues for discussion and intervention. Likewise, a reasonable hypothesis for future research is that the marginalization of contextual issues may be inversely related to patient satisfaction, an important outcome of care,[5] and that for many patients more explicit attention to contextual problems would enhance satisfaction. Even from the standpoint of utilization and cost, it can be argued that attention to contextual concerns in many instances can improve functional status, decrease unnecessary utilization, and possibly reduce the costs of care, especially for at-risk people such as the elderly and those affected by poverty. Aiming toward a more supportive and humanistic encounter, one that can address contextual concerns rather than simply marginalizing them, may then emerge as a goal that even some enlightened managed care organizations could support.

As a fourth criterion, practitioners should consider referral to social workers, psychologists, or psychiatrists but also should evaluate whether specific patients would benefit more from dealing with contextual issues exclusively in the primary care setting. In managed care, the primary care practitioner usually initiates such referrals, but administrative reviewers, often through utilization review committees, must approve the referrals for reimbursement. For some patients, experiences with mental health professionals prove unsatisfactory or financially prohibitive. In addition, mental health professionals' role in mediating socially caused distress has received criticism both outside and inside the psychiatric profession.[6] Even aside from utilization review, because many patients do not feel comfortable seeking help from mental health professionals, primary care practitioners rather than psychiatrists probably will continue to see the majority of patients with emotional problems who present to physicians for care.[7] While referrals to mental health professionals sometimes may prove necessary or appropriate, a broad mandate encouraging such care for people suffering from contextually based distress is not a solution.

As a fifth criterion, physicians and managed care organizations should try to avoid the "medicalization" of social problems that require long-term reforms in social policy, and medicalization itself requires further critical attention.[8] At the individual level, medicalization can become a subtle process. For instance, there is a fine line between physicians' discussing contextual interventions and assuming professional control over broad arenas of patients' lives. Here it is important that physicians not imply that the solution of contextual difficulties ultimately becomes an individual's responsibility.

Clearly, it would be helpful if patients and physicians could turn to more readily available forms of assistance outside the medical arena to help in the solution of social problems, and current conditions do not evoke optimism about broader changes in medicine's social context. Such changes will require time and financial resources, although not necessarily more than those now consumed in inefficient conversations that marginalize contextual issues. Contextual problems warrant social policies to address unmet needs, and some other countries have gone far beyond the United States in enacting such policies.[9] These suggestions are not new. Yet it is evident that meaningful improvements in medical encounters will depend partly on such wider reforms that go beyond the changes inherent in managed care.

## MEDICOPOLITICAL STRUGGLE AND THE PATIENT–DOCTOR RELATIONSHIP

As managed care works its transformation of the patient–doctor relationship, the questions of consent and acquiescence present themselves. Why do patients and physicians put up with such a fundamental shift in the historical basis of their relationships? Do patients see little space to resist a new system in which physicians—the professionals with whom they previously valued close and trusting relationships, even if those relationships sometimes became flawed—have become double agents, gatekeepers who purportedly represent the interests of both patients and corporations, while corporate revenues depend in large part on restricting services? Has physicians' quest to maintain their livelihoods become so desperate that they have become, as some have argued whimsically, like lemmings marching into the sea of managed care?

Resistance among patients has mounted, although slowly. In many states, consumers' organizations have initiated campaigns to counter some of the observed excesses of managed care. These efforts have led to state-level lobbying activities for protective legislation prohibiting unreasonable limitations and delays in services. Some advocacy groups also have heavily criticized the gag rules and similar restrictions on information, by which physicians either formally or informally feel restrained from advising patients about the full range of diagnostic and therapeutic options available. As noted in chapter 4, some of this advocacy work has culminated in class-action lawsuits and similar forms of legal action that may lead to reforms in some of the constraining policies that managed care has imposed on the patient–doctor relationship.

Physicians' resistance also is gradually increasing, despite the surprising acquiescence shown so far in accepting administrative control and micromanagement of the everyday conditions of practice. State medical associations and the American Medical Association have supported legislative efforts to curb gag rules and other constraints on free communication between patients and physicians. Some physicians, both individually and in groups, have severed their contracts with managed care organizations in protest, with financial results that have varied from success to bankruptcy. A small number of new organizations have emerged, including unions, to improve physicians' bargaining position with managed care organizations and insurance companies. Such efforts, however, so far have proven surprising mild, with little criticism of the underlying structural features of managed care, especially related to its corporatization, that impinge on the patient–doctor relationship.

An important exception to passivity among U.S. physicians involves the organization that has worked to achieve a national health program for the United States. As described in chapter 7, Physicians for a National Health Program (PNHP), with chapters in all 50 states, has initiated a series of proposals that have called for a national health policy based on a single-payer approach.[10] Modeled on the Canadian system but advocating policies to correct problems that have arisen in Canada, PNHP's proposals led to the most widely supported alternative to the managed care proposal of the Clinton administration. Although congressional legislation based on the single-payer model failed along with the Clinton plan, PNHP has continued to work actively at the national and state levels to maintain the vision of a well-organized national program as a viable policy option.

One component of PNHP's work since the failure of the Clinton proposal has involved a continuing, sharp critique of managed care's impact on the patient–doctor relationship. PNHP leaders have called attention in many forums to the deleterious effects of gag rules and other restrictions on free communication between patients and physicians.[11] These efforts have contributed to movement in state legislatures and in the national Congress toward reforms that modify such practices.

A major part of this work has focused on administrative waste and the erroneous view that physicians' practice patterns account for most of the problem of high costs in health care. Although uncontrolled costs constitute a multifaceted problem, administrative waste deserves special emphasis from this viewpoint.[12] Many of the structural problems that affect the patient–doctor relationship under managed care are connected to intensive administrative practices that encourage micromanagement of clinical decisions by nonclinical administrators within insurance companies and managed care organizations.

Administrators represent the fastest-growing sector of the health care labor force, having expanded at three times the rate of physicians and other clinical personnel. Even before the latest proliferation of managed care, the United States spent more on administration than any other economically developed country: approximately 25 percent of health care costs. Countries with national health programs spend between 6 and 14 percent of health care costs on administration. A national health program that reduced administrative spending to a similar proportion would produce enough savings to provide universal access to health services without additional spending.[13]

Part of the savings achieved through a national health program could be used to address problems in the patient–doctor relationship, such as the development of systems to help deal with the contextual issues that impinge on medical encounters. Yet because managed care is administratively intensive, it tends to increase administrative expenditures, as opposed to expenditures for clinical services, even further. Administrative practices that curtail services and constrain communication in the patient–doctor relationship under managed care themselves are costly. The evidence that these added administrative costs can be justified by appropriate reductions in clinical costs has been quite limited.[14]

Inappropriate physician practices account for a small part of this country's cost crisis, in comparison with unnecessary administrative waste.[15] Overall expenditures on unnecessary procedures ordered or performed by physicians are currently unknown. Even generous estimates, however, put this figure at no more than about 10 percent of total spending on health care, a much smaller proportion than that attributed to administrative waste.[16] Under the circumstances of managed care's unproven effects in improving efficacy or reducing overall costs, the micromanagement policies that restrict clinical decisions and physicians' open explanations of them deserve greater critical attention than they have received thus far.

### TRAUMA, SOMATIZATION, AND NARRATIVE

Regarding treatment of somatoform symptoms in primary care settings, as described in chapter 5, an alliance between provider and patient has to recognize the interrelationships among trauma, somatization, culture, and narrative. In this alliance, a principal goal is the patient's feeling of safety. Frequently, refugees and immigrants have lost basic trust in institutions as a result of their previous traumatic experiences. Conditions encountered in exile may impede recovery from premigration trauma. Local violence generated by youth gangs, drug abuse and traffic, physical and sexual abuse, fear of immigration officials (which affects not only undocumented individuals, but also those with temporary visas), police brutality, lack of access to health services, and other forms of ongoing severe stress may reactivate patients' previous trauma and exacerbate physical and emotional symptoms.[17] Somatizing patients from diverse cultural backgrounds may respond to different therapeutic interventions, including group treatment and participation by culturally sensitive mental health professionals.[18]

Unfortunately, however, the most effective approach to treating somatizing patients remains unclear. Such patients, who usually present to primary care practitioners, often receive extended and expensive diagnostic evaluations, either because the physician does not recognize somatization or because he or she feels the need to exclude organic causes as well. Even when a practitioner diagnoses somatization accurately, treatment options remain limited, partly because patients often resist psychiatric evaluation and therapy.

Still, at least among the high proportion of somatizing patients who have experienced severe trauma, there is little question that bringing to consciousness a narrative of trauma, its relation to somatic symptoms, and the impact of culture at least offers promise as a treatment option to be evaluated. Although this promise is tempered by the consistent observation that ongoing economic, political, and familial issues play an important role in somatization and its treatment, therapeutic approaches that emphasize the construction of coherent narratives of trauma deserve assessment for many patients who suffer from somatoform symptoms.

Work in several fields suggests the possible value of therapeutic strategies that emphasize the formulation of coherent narratives in dealing with severe trauma.[19] For instance, psychotherapeutic explorations with survivors of childhood abuse or political trauma such as torture during adulthood suggest the importance of a patient's enunciating a coherent narrative, sometimes referred to as a "testimony," as a critical component of the healing process. Case reports of such testimonies, either in individual therapy or in nonprofessional support groups, indicate the usefulness of narratives that link trauma, culture, and physical symptoms in the treatment of patients who suffer from somatization. Such efforts cohere with findings in psychological research that "putting stress into words" not only alleviates emotional suffering, but also exerts favorable effects on physiological measures of arousal.[20]

Several colleagues and I are exploring the efficacy of Paulo Freire's model of consciousness-raising groups, which previously have been used as a technique of empowerment for educational interventions in Latin America.[21] Such techniques have achieved success in such areas as public health education and the modification of high-risk sexual behavior in AIDS control programs.[22] The techniques resemble the group processes that have provided forums for the "testimonies" of trauma victims.[23] Although empowered speech clearly is not equivalent to empowered action, several of these programs that have applied Freire's educational approaches to health care have found that many participants in empowerment groups eventually take greater initiative in dealing with adverse conditions in other arenas, such as housing and employment.[24] We are trying to study how the processing of narratives occurs in such groups and how the therapeutic (or, as Freire would say, "liberating") process might take place.

Specifically, can such groups provide a culturally sanctioned space in which the terrible narrative finally could be returned to consciousness, expressed explicitly and coherently, and worked through in a supportive social context? Although this question has not yet been answered, intervention studies that evaluate and compare empowerment groups versus other therapeutic options for somatizing patients will clarify the efficacy of approaches encouraging the expression of coherent narratives that link trauma, culture, and somatoform symptoms. This conceptual approach to narratives of trauma and somatization may prove therapeutically more useful than the current tendency to deal with extreme stress in a manner that, though culturally sanctioned, becomes expensive, misleading, and perhaps more painful somatically than need be the case.

## STILL "WAITING FOR LEFTY"

During the Great Depression, the playwright Clifford Odets captured some key themes that I have tried to develop more than 60 years later. In *Waiting for Lefty*, Dr. Benjamin—a medical resident at a large urban hospital—tries to diagnose and treat his patients supportively.[25] But he finds that broader social problems constrain his relationships with patients. Dealing with a financial deficit, the hospital's board of directors decides to close another charity ward, where low-income patients previously could receive urgent services at reduced cost. "Benj" learns, influenced partly by his teacher, Barnes, that financial considerations govern the policies that affect not only the hospital, but the larger health care system of which it is a part.

As he becomes more dispirited about the possibilities for humane relationships with his patients, Benj reads about what appear to be more favorable possibilities under socialized medicine in the Soviet Union. He fantasizes that there, his capabilities as a healer could be fulfilled with less social impediment.

At the end, though, Benj opts to struggle within the United States. He enters political work in his few free hours. Although he commits himself to this struggle, he also recognizes his own apprehension about the difficulties and uncertainties involved: "No! Our work's here—America! I'm scared. . . . What future's ahead, I don't know."

Those who follow at the front lines of medicine at the start of a new millennium still are waiting, struggling, scared, hopeful.

# appendix

◆ ◆

Groups in Latin American Social Medicine That Conduct
Research on the Social Determinants of Health

| Country | Group | Leaders | Foci | Comments |
|---|---|---|---|---|
| Argentina | Buenos Aires | Mario Testa, Celia Iriart, Laura Nervi, Francisco Leone, Silvia Faraone | strategic planning, history of public health, health policy, environmental health, mental health | courses at University of Buenos Aires; collaborations with labor unions |
| | Buenos Aires | José Carlos Escudero, Enrique Kreplak, Matilde Ruderman, Alicia Stolkiner, Marcos Buchbinder, Deborah Tajer, Liliana Mayoral | environmental health, mental health, health policy, research methods | journal, *Salud, Problema y Debate*; help coordinate Latin American Association of Social Medicine |
| | Rosario | Carlos Bloch, Susana Belmartino, Irene Luppi, Zulema Quinteros, María del Carmen Troncoso | medical profession, social epidemiology, health policy | research center: Centro de Estudios Sanitarios y Sociales; journal, *Cuadernos Médico Sociales* |
| | Córdoba | Horacio Barri, Norma Fernández, Sylvia Bermann, Héctor Seia | medical education, occupational health, community-based epidemiology, health communication | maintain values of Movement for an Integral Health System; journal, *Salud y Sociedad*; collaborate with labor unions |
| Brazil | | | | "collective health"; influence of theology of liberation and empowerment education; national organization: *Asociación Brasiliera de Pós-Graduação em Saúde Colectiva* |

| Brazil | São Paulo | María Cecilia Donnangelo, Ricardo Bruno Mendes Gonçalves, Amelia Cohn, Paulo Elias, Lilia Shraiber, José Ricardo Ayres, Paulette Goldemberg, Rita Baradas Barrata | work process in health, economic policies, medical education, philosophy of epidemiology | collaborations with Workers Party |
|---|---|---|---|---|
| | Campinas | Emerson Merhy, Gastão Wagner de Sousa Campos, Everardo Duarte Nunes | health policy and planning, history of public health, health administration, microlevel processes | Laboratory of Administration and Planning; collaborations with municipal and state governments, labor unions, Workers Party; journal, *Saúde em Debate* |
| | Rio de Janeiro | Sergio Arouca, Paulo Buss, Hesio Cordeiro, Madel Luz, Sonia Fleury, Cristina Possas | health policy, critical epidemiology, institutional analysis | importance of Oswaldo Cruz Foundation, National School of Public Health; journal, *Cadernos de Saúde Pública* |
| | Bahía | Naomar de Almeida Filho, Sebastian Loureiro, Carmen Fontes Teixeira, Jairnilson Paim, Mauricio Lima Barreto | multimethod epidemiology, public health planning | epidemiological teaching, conferences |
| Chile | Santiago | Alfredo Estrada, Adriana Vega, Jaime Sepúlveda, Carlos Montoya, Mariano Requena, Marilú Soto, Enrique Barilari, Silvia Riquelme, Felipe Cabello, Hugo Behm | mental health, gender and health, occupational and environmental health, social epidemiology, health policy | research and training center: Grupo de Investigación y Capacitación en Medicina Social; journal, *Salud y Cambio* |

| Country | Group | Leaders | Foci | Comments |
|---|---|---|---|---|
| Colombia | Bogotá, Medellín, Cali | Saúl Franco, Alberto Vasco | urban poverty and marginalization, infectious diseases, occupational health, gender, violence, social class | affected by recurrent violence |
| Cuba | Havana | Francisco Rojas Ochoa, Cosmé Ordóñez, Silvia Martínez Calvo | history of social medicine, community-oriented medical education, geriatric medicine, interface with primary care | debate about need for social medicine; journal, *Boletín de Ateneo Juan César García* |
| Ecuador | Quito | Jaime Breilh, Arturo Campaña, Oscar Betancourt, Edmundo Granda, Francisco Hidalgo | critical epidemiology, multimethod research, work process, gender, mental health, health policy | research and consulting center: Centro de Estudios y Asesoría en Salud; work with national coalition |
| Mexico | Mexico City, Guadalajara | Asa Cristina Laurell, Catalina Eibenschutz, Carolina Tetelboin, Mariano Noriega, José Blanco Gil, Oliva López, Eduardo Menéndez, Francisco Mercado | occupational health, community health, multimethod and participatory research, health policy | graduate program, Autonomous Metropolitan University; journal, *Salud Problema*; collaborations with labor unions, Revolutionary Democratic Party, Zapatista Army for National Liberation |

*Source:* H. Waitzkin, C. Iriart, A. Estrada, and S. Lamadrid, "Social Medicine in Latin America," *Lancet* 358(2001): 315–23.

# notes

◆ ◆

CHAPTER ONE

1. A. Fine, "Care denials causing a stir among physicians," *Executive Solutions Healthcare Management* 11(1999): 2–5; C.M. Fagin and S. Gordon, "The abandonment of the patient," *Nursing Outlook* 3(1996): 147–49; P. Spath, "Managed care resurrects 'dumping' fears," *Hospital Peer Review* 7(1997): 17, 20–25.

2. *Undocumented Migration to the United States: IRCA and the Experience of the 1980s*, ed. F.D. Bean, B. Edmonston, and J.S. Passel (Washington, DC: Urban Institute Press, 1990); G.J. Borjas, *Friends or Strangers: The Impact of Immigrants on the U.S. Economy* (New York: Basic Books, 1990); J.L. Simon, *The Economic Consequences of Migration* (Cambridge: Basic Blackwell, 1989); M. Fix and J.S. Passel, "Immigration and immigrants: Setting the record straight," *Urban Institute* publication, May 1994; J.S. Passel and R.L. Clark, "Immigrants in New York: Their legal status, incomes, and taxes," *Urban Institute* publication, April 1998; L. Ku and B. Kessler, *The Number and Cost of Immigrants on Medicaid: National and State Estimates* (Washington, DC: Urban Institute, 1997).

3. M.L. Berk, C.L. Schur, L.R. Chavez, and M. Frankel, "Health care use among undocumented Latino immigrants," *Health Affairs* 19(2000): 51–64; F.A. Hubbell, H. Waitzkin, S.I. Mishra, J. Dombrink, and L.R. Chavez, "Access to medical care for documented and undocumented Latinos in a southern California county," *Western Journal of Medicine* 154(1991): 414–17.

4. R. Kuttner, "The American health care system: Health insurance coverage," *New England Journal of Medicine* 340(1999): 163–68; R. Kuttner, "The American health care system: Employer-sponsored health coverage," *New England Journal of Medicine* 340(1999): 248–52.

5. S. Woolhandler and D.U. Himmelstein, "The deteriorating administrative efficiency of the U.S. health care system," *New England Journal of Medicine* 324(1991): 1253–58; D.J. Shulkin, A.L. Hillman, and W.M. Cooper, "Reasons for increasing administrative costs in hospitals," *Annals of*

205

*Internal Medicine* 119(1993): 74–78; S. Woolhandler and D.U. Himmelstein, "Costs of care and administration at for-profit and other hospitals in the United States," *New England Journal of Medicine* 336(1997): 769–74.

6. For a calculation of savings through reduced administrative expenditures and the implications for a national health program, see U.S. General Accounting Office, *Canadian Health Insurance: Lessons for the United States* (Washington, DC: Government Printing Office [GAO Publ. No. GAO/HRD-91-90; B-244081], 1991).

7. H.L. Fuenzalida-Puelma, L. Hernán, and S.S. Connor, *The Right to Health in the Americas: A Comparative Constitutional Study* (Washington, DC: Pan American Health Organization, 1989).

8. For a concise statement of this viewpoint, see A. Enthoven and R. Kronick, "Universal health insurance through incentives reform," *JAMA* 265(1991): 2532–36.

9. T.S. Snail and J.C. Robinson, "Organizational diversification in the American hospital," *Annual Review of Public Health* 19(1998): 417–53; J.C. Robinson, "Decline in hospital utilization and cost inflation under managed care in California," *JAMA* 276(1996): 1060–64; J.C. Robinson, "The dynamics and limits of corporate growth in health care," *Health Affairs* 15(1996): 155–69; J.C. Robinson and L.B. Gardner, "Adverse selection among multiple competing health maintenance organizations," *Medical Care* 33(1995): 1161–75.

10. J. Holahan, S. Zuckerman, A. Evans, and S. Rangarajan, "Medicaid managed care in thirteen states," *Health Affairs* 17(1998): 43–63.; R.T. Slifkin, S.D. Hoag, P. Silberman, S. Felt-Lisk, and B. Popkin, "Medicaid managed care programs in rural areas: A fifty-state overview," *Health Affairs* 17(1998): 217–27; M. Gold and A. Aizer, "Growing an industry: How managed is TennCare's managed care?" *Health Affairs* 19(2000): 86–101.

11. B.H. Gray, *The Profit Motive and Patient Care* (Cambridge, MA: Harvard University Press, 1991); B.H. Gray, "Ownership matters: Health reform and the future of nonprofit health care," *Inquiry* 30(1993): 352–61; B.H. Gray, "Conversion of HMOs and hospitals: What's at stake?" *Health Affairs* 16(1997): 29–47; H. Waitzkin, *The Second Sickness: Contradictions of Capitalist Health Care* (Lanham, MD: Rowman & Littlefield, 2000), 97–117.

12. *Fortune* 500, 2000 (<www.fortune.com>, September 2000).

13. D.U. Himmelstein, S. Woolhandler, I. Hellender, and S.M. Wolfe, "Quality of care in investor-owned vs. not-for-profit HMOs," *JAMA* 282(1999): 159–63; E.M. Silverman, J.S. Skinner, and E.S. Fisher, "The association between for-profit hospital ownership and increased Medicare spending," *New England Journal of Medicine* 341(1999): 420–26.

14. E. Ginzberg, H.S. Berliner, and M. Ostow, *Changing U.S. Health Care: A Study of Four Metropolitan Areas* (Boulder, CO: Westview, 1993). For more on corporate takeover of hospitals that serve indigent clients, see also chapter 6.

15. Children's Defense Fund, *The State of America's Children: Yearbook 2000* (Washington, DC: Children's Defense Fund, 2000); National Center for Health Statistics, "Infant, neonatal, and postneonatal mortality rates, according to detailed race of mother and Hispanic origin of mother: United States, 1983–91 birth cohorts," September 2000 <http://www.cdc.gov/nchs/datawh/statab/pubd/hus-t20h.htm>; *Health, United States, 1995* (Hyattsville, MD: Public Health Service, 1996), 99; S.L. Carmichael and S. Iyasu, "Changes in the black–white infant mortality gap from 1983 to 1991 in the United States," *American Journal of Preventive Medicine* 15 (1998): 220–27.

## CHAPTER TWO

1. H. Waitzkin, "Truth's search for power: The dilemmas of the social sciences," *Social Problems* 15(1968): 408–18.

2. C.E. Lewis, "Health-services research and innovations in health care delivery: Does research make a difference?" *New England Journal of Medicine* 297(1977): 423–27.

3. Waitzkin, "Truth's search for power: The dilemmas of the social sciences"; H. Waitzkin and F.A. Hubbell, "Truth's search for power: Critical applications to community-oriented primary care and small area analysis," *Medical Care Review* 49(1992): 161–89.

4. S.L. Kark, *Community-Oriented Primary Care* (New York: Appleton-Century-Crofts, 1981); S.L. Kark and J.H. Abramson, "Community-focused health care," *Israel Journal of Medical Sciences* 17(1981): 65–70; P.A. Nutting and E.M. Connor, "Community-oriented primary care: An examination of the U.S. experience," *American Journal of Public Health* 76(1986): 279–81; P.A. Nutting, M. Wood, and E.M. Connor, "Community-oriented primary care in the United States: A status report." *JAMA* 253(1985): 1763–66; R. Rhyne, R. Bogue, G. Kukulka, and H. Fulmer, eds., *Community-Oriented Primary Care: Health Care for the 21st Century* (Washington, DC: American Public Health Association, 1998).

5. Kark, *Community-Oriented Primary Care*.

6. Ibid., 194–246.

7. S.R. Benatar, "Medicine and health care in South Africa," *New England Journal of Medicine* 315(1986): 527–32; R.W. Turton and B.E. Chalmers, "Apartheid, stress and illness: The demographic context of distress reported by South Africans," *Social Science & Medicine* 31(1990): 1191–1200; M. Turshen, "Health and human rights in a South African Bantustan," *Social Science & Medicine* 22(1986): 887–92.

8. Kark, *Community-Oriented Primary Care*, 91–193; Turton and Chalmers, "Apartheid, stress and illness."

9. R.L. Punamaki and R. Suleiman, "Predictors and effectiveness of coping with political violence among Palestinian children," *British Journal of Social Psychology* 29(1990): 67–77; N. Reiss, "The health care of Arabs in

Israel," *Journal of Palestinian Studies*, 22(1993): 73–93; R.H.B. Fishman, "War of words continues over Palestinian health care," *Lancet* 350(1997): 1527.

10. Institute of Medicine, *Community-Oriented Primary Care: A Practical Assessment*, vol. 1 (Washington, DC: National Academy Press, 1984); Rhyne, Bogue, Kukulka, and Fulmer, *Community-Oriented Primary Care.*

11. D.E. Rogers, "Community-oriented primary care," *JAMA* 248(1982): 1622–25.

12. P.A. Nutting, ed., *Community-Oriented Primary Care: From Principle to Practice* (Washington, DC: U.S. Department of Health and Human Services [Health Resources and Services Administration Publication No. HRS-A-PE 86-1], 1987); Rhyne, Bogue, Kukulka, and Fulmer, *Community-Oriented Primary Care.*

13. Rhyne, Bogue, Kukulka, and Fulmer, *Community-Oriented Primary Care.*

14. Waitzkin, *The Second Sickness*, 97–117.

15. J.E. Wennberg, J.L. Freeman, and W.J. Culp, "Are hospital services rationed in New Haven or over-utilised in Boston?" *Lancet* 1(1987): 1185–89; R.H. Brook, "Practice guidelines and practicing medicine: Are they compatible?" *JAMA* 262(1989): 3027–30; Dartmouth Medical School, Center for the Evaluative Clinical Sciences, *The Dartmouth Atlas of Health Care* (Chicago: American Hospital Publishing, 1998). For overviews and collections of practice guidelines, see <www.ahrq.gov> (September 2000).

16. For research on variations in practice patterns, see Dartmouth Medical School, *The Dartmouth Atlas of Health Care*; G.T. O'Connor, H.B. Quinton, N.D. Traven, L.D. Ramunno, T.A. Dodds, T.A. Marciniak, and J.E. Wennberg, "Geographic variation in the treatment of acute myocardial infarction: The Cooperative Cardiovascular Project," *JAMA* 281 (1999): 627–33; J.E. Wennberg, "Understanding geographic variations in health care delivery," *New England Journal of Medicine* 340(1999): 52–53; J.D. Birkmeyer, S.M. Sharp, S.R. Finlayson, E.S. Fisher, and J.E. Wennberg, "Variation profiles of common surgical procedures," *Surgery* 124(1998): 917–23.

17. E. Freidson, *Profession of Medicine* (Chicago: University of Chicago Press, 1988); D.J. Hyman and V.N. Pavlik, "Self-reported hypertension treatment practices among primary care physicians: Blood pressure thresholds, drug choices, and the role of guidelines and evidence-based medicine," *Archives of Internal Medicine* 160(2000): 2281–86; R. Grilli, N. Magrini, A. Penna, G. Mura, and A. Liberati, "Practice guidelines developed by specialty societies: The need for a critical appraisal," *Lancet* 355(2000): 103–6; L. Gundersen, "The effect of clinical practice guidelines on variations in care," *Annals of Internal Medicine* 133(2000): 317–18; J.M. Spandorfer, Y. Israel, and B.J. Turner, "Primary care physicians' views on screening and management of alcohol abuse: Inconsistencies with national guidelines," *Journal of Family Practice* 48(1999): 899–902; M.D. Cabana, C.S. Rand, N.R. Powe, A.W. Wu, M.H. Wilson, P.A. Abboud, and

H.R. Rubin, "Why don't physicians follow clinical practice guidelines? A framework for improvement," *JAMA* 282(1999): 1458–65.

18. For a classic analysis of this issue that has maintained its relevance, see National Leadership Commission on Health Care, *For the Health of a Nation*, Technical Appendix III (Washington, DC: National Leadership Commission on Health Care, 1989).

19. For examples illustrating this type of research, see J. Billings, L. Zeitel, J. Lukomnik, T.S. Carey, A.E. Blank, and L. Newman, "Impact of socioeconomic status on hospital use in New York City," *Health Affairs* 12(1)(1993): 162–73; H. Krakauer, I. Jacoby, M. Millman, and J.E. Lukomnik, "Physician impact on hospital admission and on mortality rates in the Medicare population," *Health Services Research* 31(1996): 191–211; N.R. Powe, J.P. Weiner, B. Starfield, M. Stuart, A. Baker, and D.M. Steinwachs, "Systemwide provider performance in a Medicaid program: Profiling the care of patients with chronic illnesses," *Medical Care* 34(1996): 798–810; American College of Obstetricians and Gynecologists, "Ambulatory care sensitive indication: Ectopic pregnancy, ruptured," *International Journal of Gynaecology and Obstetrics* 57(1997): 229–30.

20. For examples of such local, anthropologically oriented research on access and health policy issues, see A. Dill, "Institutional environments and organizational responses to AIDS," *Journal of Health & Social Behavior* 35(1994): 349–69; H. Waitzkin, R.L. Williams, J.A. Bock, and J. McCloskey, "Impacts of Medicaid managed care on low-income persons and safety-net providers in a rural state: A multimethod assessment," *American Journal of Public Health* (2001, in press); S. Horton, M. Henriksen, J. McCloskey, T. Thomas, and C. Todd, "Transforming the safety net: Medicaid managed care in rural and urban New Mexico," *American Anthropologist* (2001, in press).

## CHAPTER THREE

1. Early works that considered the social origins of illness, but with a different analytic perspective, include G. Rosen, "What is social medicine?" *Bulletin of the History of Medicine* 21(1947): 674–733; G. Rosen, *A History of Public Health* (New York: MD Publications, 1958), especially 192–293; R. Sand, *The Advance to Social Medicine* (London: Staples Press, 1952), especially 295–343, 507–89; H. E. Sigerist, *Civilization and Disease* (Ithaca, NY: Cornell University Press, 1944), 6–64. For a more extensive discussion of this history, see Waitzkin, *The Second Sickness*, 55–73; H. Waitzkin, C. Iriart, A. Estrada, and S. Lamadrid, "Social medicine in Latin America," *Lancet* 358(2001): 315–23; and H. Waitzkin, C. Iriart, A. Estrada, and S. Lamadrid, "Social medicine then and now: Lessons from Latin America," *American Journal of Public Health* (2001, in press).

2. F. Engels, *The Condition of the Working Class in England in 1844* (Moscow: Progress Publishers, 1973 [1845]).

3. For a sympathetic critique, see S. Marcus, *Engels, Manchester, and the Working Class* (New York: Vintage, 1974).

4. Engels, *The Condition of the Working Class in England in 1844*, 135.

5. E. Chadwick, *Inquiry into the Sanitary Condition of the Labouring Population of Great Britain* (Edinburgh: Edinburgh University Press, 1965 [1842]), especially 80–254.

6. Engels, *The Condition of the Working Class in England in 1844*, 141–42.

7. Ibid., 142–43.

8. Ibid., 190–93.

9. Ibid., 230.

10. Ibid., 200.

11. Ibid., 279–84.

12. F. Engels, *Herr Eugen Dühring's Revolution in Science [Anti-Dühring]* (New York: International, 1966 [1878]); F. Engels, *Dialectics of Nature* (New York: International, 1940).

13. R. Virchow, *Cellular Pathology* (New York: De Witt, 1860).

14. R. Virchow, *Disease, Life, and Man*, trans. L. J. Rather (Stanford, CA: Stanford University Press, 1958), 27–29. Unless otherwise noted, I have prepared the translations from German and Spanish.

15. E.H. Ackerknecht, *Rudolf Virchow: Doctor, Statesman, Anthropologist* (Madison: University of Wisconsin Press, 1953), 52.

16. Virchow, *Disease, Life, and Man*, 142–50.

17. R. Virchow, *Werk und Wirkung* (Berlin: Rütten & Loenig, 1957), 94–96.

18. R. Virchow, *Gesammelte Abhandlungen aus dem Gebiet der Öffentlichen Medicin und der Seuchenlehre*, vol. 1 (Berlin: Hirschwald, 1879), 305, 321–34.

19. Virchow, *Werk und Wirkung*, 42, 104.

20. Virchow, *Gesammelte Abhandlungen*, vol. 1, 121–22; Ackerknecht, *Rudolf Virchow*, 125–29.

21. Virchow, *Werk und Wirkung*, 110.

22. Ibid., 55; Ackerknecht, *Rudolf Virchow*, 131–38.

23. Virchow, *Werk und Wirkung*, 108, 127.

24. Ibid., 106.

25. Ibid., 117; Virchow, *Disease, Life, and Man*, 106.

26. J.C. Escudero,"El impacto epidemiológico de la invasión europea a américa," *Salud y Cambio* (Chile) 3(7)(1992): 4–11; E. Galeano, *Open Veins of Latin America* (New York: Monthly Review Press, 1997).

27. M. Foucault, "El nacimiento de la medicina social," *Revista Centroamericana de Ciencias de la Salud* 3(6)(1977): 89–108; G. Rosen, *De la Política Médica a la Medicina Social* (Mexico City, Mexico: Siglo XXI, 1985).

28. E.D. Nunes, "Trayectoría de la medicina social en América Latina: elementos para su configuración," in *Debates en Medicina Social*, ed. S. Franco, E.D. Nunes, J. Breilh, and C. Laurell (Quito, Ecuador: Organización Panamericana de la Salud/ALAMES, 1991).

29. A. Flexner, *Medical Education in the United States and Canada* (New York: Arno Press, 1972 [1910]).

30. E.R. Brown, *Rockefeller Medicine Men* (Berkeley: University of California Press, 1979).

31. M.A. Illanes, *"En el Nombre del Pueblo, del Estado y de la Ciencia, . . .":* *Historia Social de la Salud Pública, Chile 1880–1973* (Santiago, Chile: Colectivo de Atención Primaria, 1993).

32. E. Cruz-Coke, *Medicina Preventiva y Medicina Dirigida* (Santiago, Chile: Editorial Nascimento, 1938).

33. S. Allende, *La Realidad Médico-Social Chilena* (Santiago, Chile: Ministerio de Salubridad, Previsión y Asistencia Social, 1939).

34. Ibid., 6, 8.

35. Ibid., 86.

36. Ibid., 105.

37. Ibid., 119.

38. Ibid., 124.

39. Ibid., 189–90.

40. Ibid., 191.

41. Ibid., 198.

42. H. Waitzkin, "Is our work dangerous? Should it be?" *Journal of Health and Social Behavior* 39(1998): 7–17; H. Waitzkin, C. Iriart, A. Estrada, and S. Lamadrid, "Social medicine in Latin America," *Lancet* 358(2001): 315–23.

43. Engels, *Dialectics of Nature*; R. Levins and R. Lewontin, *The Dialectical Biologist* (Cambridge, MA: Harvard University Press, 1985).

44. A.C. Laurell, "La salud-enfermedad como proceso social," *Revista Latinoamericana de Salud* (Mexico City) 2(1982): 7–25; S. Franco, "La cuestión de la causalidad en medicina," in Grupo de Trabajo, *Desarrollo de la Medicina Social en America Latina, OPS-ALAMES* (Mexico City: Organización Panamericana de la Salud, 1989).

45. M. Marmot and A. Feeney, "General explanations for social inequalities and health," *IARC Scientific Publications* (Lyon), 138(1997): 207–28; P. Martikainen, S. Stansfeld, H. Hemingway, and M. Marmot, "Determinants of socioeconomic differences in change in physical and mental functioning," *Social Science & Medicine* 49(1999): 499–507; M.G. Marmot, R. Fuhrer, S.L. Ettner, N.F. Marks, L.L. Bumpass, and C.D. Ryff, "Contribution of psychosocial factors to socioeconomic differences in health," *Milbank Quarterly* 76(1998): 403–48.

46. G.A. Kaplan, E. Pamuk, J.W. Lynch, R.D. Cohen, and J.L. Balfour, "Inequality in income and mortality in the United States: Analysis of mortality and potential pathways," *BMJ* 312(1996): 999–1003; B.P. Kennedy, I. Kawachi, and D. Prothrow-Stith, "Income distribution and mortality: Cross-sectional ecological study of the Robin Hood index in the United States," *BMJ* 312(1996): 1004–7; J. Lynch, G.A. Kaplan, E.R. Pamuk, R.D. Cohen, K.E. Heck, J.L. Balfour, and I.H. Yen, "Income inequality and mortality in metropolitan areas of the United States," *American Journal of Public Health* 88(1998): 1074–80; L. M. Schalick, W.C. Hadden, E. Pamuk, V.

Navarro, and G. Pappas, "The widening gap in death rates among income groups in the United States from 1967 to 1986," *International Journal of Health Services* 30(2000): 13–26; J.W. Lynch, G.D. Smith, G.A. Kaplan, and J.S. House, "Income inequality and mortality: Importance to health of individual income, psychosocial environment, or material conditions," *BMJ* 320(2000): 1200–1204.

47. R.G. Wilkinson, *Unhealthy Societies: The Afflictions of Inequality* (London: Routledge, 1996); I. Kawachi, B. Kennedy, and R.G. Wilkinson, eds., *Income Inequality and Health: A Reader* (New York: New Press, 1999).

48. A.V. Diez-Roux, B. Link, and M.E. Northridge, "A multilevel analysis of income inequality and cardiovascular disease risk factors," *Social Science & Medicine* 50(2000): 73–87; A.V. Diez-Roux, "Multilevel analysis in public health research," *Annual Review of Public Health* 21(2000): 171–92; B.P. Kennedy, I. Kawachi, D. Prothrow-Stith, K. Lochner, and B. Gibbs, "Income distribution, socioeconomic status, and self-rated health: A U.S. multilevel analysis," *BMJ* 317(1998): 917–21.

49. C. McCord and H.P. Freeman, "Excess mortality in Harlem," *New England Journal of Medicine* 322(1990): 1606–7; A.T. Geronimus, J. Bound, T.A. Waidmann, M.M. Hillemeier, and P.B. Burns, "Excess mortality among blacks and whites in the United States," *New England Journal of Medicine* 335(1996): 1552–58; J. Fang, S. Madhaven, and M.H. Alderman, "The association between birthplace and mortality from cardiovascular causes among black and white residents of New York City," *New England Journal of Medicine* 335(1996): 1545–51; National Center for Health Statistics, *Health, United States, 1999, with Health and Aging Chartbook* (Hyattsville, MD: National Center for Health Statistics, 1999), 30; National Center for Health Statistics, *Health, United States, 2000 with Adolescent Health Chartbook* (Hyattsville, MD: National Center for Health Statistics, 2000), 7.

50. S.L. Carmichael and S. Iyasu, "Changes in the black–white infant mortality gap from 1983 to 1991 in the United States," *American Journal of Preventive Medicine* 15(1998): 220–27; S.L. Carmichael, S. Iyasu, and K. Hatfield-Timajchy, "Cause-specific trends in neonatal mortality among black and white infants, United States, 1980–1995," *Maternal & Child Health Journal* 2(1998): 67–76; National Center for Health Statistics, *Health, United States, 2000*, 8.

51. K.A. Schulman, J.A. Berlin, W. Harless et al., "The effect of race and sex on physicians' recommendations for cardiac catheterization," *New England Journal of Medicine* 380(1999): 618–26.

52. B.P. Kennedy, I. Kawachi, K. Lochner, C.P. Jones, and D. Prothrow-Stith, "(Dis)respect and black mortality," *Ethnicity & Disease* 7(1997): 207–14.

53. D.R. Williams, "The monitoring of racial/ethnic status in the USA: Data quality issues," *Ethnicity & Health* 4(1999): 121–37; D.R. Williams, "Race, socioeconomic status, and health: The added effects of racism and

discrimination," *Annals of the New York Academy of Sciences* 896(1999): 173–88; X.S. Ren, B.C. Amick, and D.R. Williams, "Racial/ethnic disparities in health: The interplay between discrimination and socioeconomic status," *Ethnicity & Disease* 9(1999): 151–65; D.R. Williams, "Race and health: Basic questions, emerging directions," *Annals of Epidemiology* 7(1997): 322–33.

54. For an overview of this literature on gender bias in diagnosis and treatment, see V. Elderkin-Thompson and H. Waitzkin, "Difficulties in clinical communication with female patients: Are there diagnostic and treatment implications?" *Journal of General Internal Medicine* 14(1999): 112–21.

55. P. McDonough, D.R. Williams, J.S. House, and G.J. Duncan, "Gender and the socioeconomic gradient in mortality," *Journal of Health & Social Behavior* 40(1999): 17–31; S.S. Rathore, A.K. Berger, K.P. Weinfurt et al., "Race, sex, poverty, and the medical treatment of acute myocardial infarction in the elderly," *Circulation* 102(2000): 642–48; S.E. Sheifer, J.J. Escarce, and K.A. Schulman, "Race and sex differences in the management of coronary artery disease," *American Heart Journal* 139(2000): 848–57; J.S. Mandelblatt, J. Hadley, J.F. Kerner et al., "Patterns of breast carcinoma treatment in older women: Patient preference and clinical and physical influences," *Cancer* 89(2000): 561–73; J.S. Mandelblatt, K.R. Yabroff, and J.F. Kerner, "Equitable access to cancer services: A review of barriers to quality care," *Cancer* 86(1999): 2378–90; J.S. Mandelblatt, K. Gold, A.S. O'Malley et al., "Breast and cervix cancer screening among multiethnic women: Role of age, health, and source of care," *Preventive Medicine* 28(1999): 418–25.

56. R.G. Wilkinson, "Putting the picture together: Prosperity, redistribution, health, and welfare," in M. Marmot and R.G. Wikinson, eds., *Social Determinants of Health* (Oxford: Oxford University Press, 1999), 256–74; I. Kawachi, B.P. Kennedy, V. Gupta, and D. Prothrow-Stith, "Women's status and the health of women: A view from the States," *Social Science & Medicine* 48(1999): 21–32.

57. I. Kawachi, B.P. Kennedy, K. Lochner, and D. Prothrow-Stith, "Social capital, income inequality and mortality," *American Journal of Public Health* 87(1997): 1491–98; B. Kennedy, I. Kawachi, D. Prothrow-Stith, K. Lochner, and B. Gibbs, "Social capital, income inequality, and firearm violent crime," *Social Science & Medicine* 47(1998): 7–17. For more on the concept of social capital, see J.S. Coleman, "Social capital in the creation of human capital," *American Journal of Sociology* 94(supp.) (1988): S95–S120; S. Baron, J. Field, and T. Schuller, *Social Capital: Critical Perspectives* (New York: Oxford University Press, 2001); R.D. Putnam, *Bowling Alone: The Collapse and Revival of American Community* (New York: Simon & Schuster, 2000).

58. M.G. Marmot, D.S. George, S. Standsfeld et al., "Health inequalities among British civil servants: The Whitehall II study," *Lancet* 337(1991): 1387–93; C.T. van Rossum, M.J. Shipley, H. van de Mheen, D.E. Grobbee,

and M.G. Marmot, "Employment grade differences in cause specific mortality: A 25 year follow up of civil servants from the first Whitehall study," *Journal of Epidemiology & Community Health* 54(2000): 178–84.

59. World Health Organization, *Basic Health Statistics, 1999* <http://www.who.int./whosis/hfa/countries/can4.htm>; D.L. Williamson and J.E. Fast, "Poverty and medical treatment: When public policy compromises accessibility," *Canadian Journal of Public Health* 89(1998): 120–24; C.M. Bell, M. Crystal, A.S. Detsky, and D.A. Redelmeier, "Shopping around for hospital services: A comparison of the United States and Canada," *JAMA* 279(1998): 1015–17; S.J. Katz, C. Charles, J. Lomas, and H.G. Welch, "Physician relations in Canada: Shooting inward as the circle closes," *Journal of Health Politics, Policy and Law* 22(1997): 1413–31; S. J. Katz, T.P. Hofer, and W.G. Manning, "Hospital utilization in Ontario and the United States: The impact of socioeconomic status and health status," *Canadian Journal of Public Health* 87(1996): 253–56.

60. For instance: J.D. Wark, "Osteoporosis: A global perspective," *Bulletin of the World Health Organization* 77(1999): 424–26; "Cervical cancer in developing countries: Memorandum from a WHO meeting," *Bulletin of the World Health Organization* 74(1996): 345–51; J.T. Boerma, K.I. Weinstein, S.O. Rustein, and A.E. Sommerfelt, "Data on birth weight in developing countries: Can surveys help?" *Bulletin of the World Health Organization* 74(1996): 209–16.

61. S. Cereseto and H. Waitzkin, "Economic development, political–economic system, and the physical quality of life," *American Journal of Public Health* 76(1986): 661–66; S. Cereseto and H. Waitzkin, "Capitalism, socialism, and the physical quality of life," *International Journal of Health Services* 16(1986): 643–58.

62. For example, see H. Waitzkin, "Health policy and social change: A comparative history of Chile and Cuba," *Social Problems* 31(1983): 235–48; H. Waitzkin, *The Politics of Medical Encounters: How Patients and Doctors Deal with Social Problems* (New Haven, CT: Yale University Press, 1991), 265–72; H. Waitzkin, K. Wald, R. Kee, R. Danielson, and L. Robinson, "Primary care in Cuba: Low- and high-technology developments pertinent to family medicine," *Journal of Family Practice* 45(1997): 250–58.

63. D.A. Barr and M.G. Field, "The current state of health care in the former Soviet Union: Implications for health care policy and reform," *American Journal of Public Health* 86(1996): 307–12; T.H. Tulchinsky and E.A. Varavikova, "Addressing the epidemiologic transition in the former Soviet Union: Strategies for health system and public health reform in Russia," *American Journal of Public Health* 86(1996): 313–20; J.B. Wyon, "Comment: Deteriorating health in Russia—a place for community-based approaches," *American Journal of Public Health* 86(1996): 321–23; F.C. Notzon, Y.M. Komarov, S.P. Ermakov et al., "Causes of declining life expectancy in Russia: Letter from Russia," *JAMA* 279(1998): 793–800; P. Walberg, M. McKee, V. Shkolnikov, and L.D. Chenet, "Economic

change, crime, and mortality crisis in Russia: Regional analysis," *British Medical Journal* 317(1998): 312–18; W.C. Cockerham, "The social determinants of the decline of life expectancy in Russia and eastern Europe: A lifestyle explanation," *Journal of Health and Social Behavior* 38(1997): 117–30; M. Boback and M. Marmot, "Alcohol and mortality in Russia: Is it different than elsewhere?" *Annals of Epidemiology* 9(1999): 335–38; M. Marmot, "Introduction," in M. Marmot and R.G. Wilkinson, eds., *Social Determinants of Health* (Oxford: Oxford University Press, 1999), 1–16; Wilkinson, *Unhealthy Societies*, 121–30; M. Marmot, "Epidemiology of socioeconomic status and health: Are determinants within countries the same as between countries?" *Annals of the New York Academy of Sciences* 896(1999): 16–29; M. Bobak, H. Pikhart, C. Hertzman, R. Rose, and M. Marmot, "Socioeconomic factors, perceived control and self-reported health in Russia: A cross-sectional survey," *Social Science & Medicine* 47(1998): 269–79.

## CHAPTER FOUR

1. A.R. Davies, J.E. Ware, Jr., R.H. Brook, J.R. Peterson, and J.P. Newhouse, "Consumer acceptance of prepaid and fee-for-service medical care: Results from a randomized controlled trial," *Health Services Research* 21(1986): 429–52; "Health care in crisis: Are HMOs the answer?" *Consumer Reports* 57(1992, August): 519–31; H.R. Rubin, B. Gandek, W.H. Rogers, M. Kosinski, C.A. McHorney, and J.E. Ware, Jr., "Patients' ratings of outpatients visits in different practice settings: Results from the Medical Outcomes Study," *JAMA* 270(1993): 835–40; D.U. Himmelstein, S. Woolhandler, I. Hellander, and S.M. Wolfe, "Quality of care in investor-owned vs. not-for-profit HMO's," *JAMA* 282(1999): 159–63; H. Waitzkin and M.A. Cook, "Managed care and the geriatric patient–physician relationship," *Clinics in Geriatric Medicine* 16(2000): 133–51.

2. M. Angell, "The doctor as double agent," *Kennedy Institute for Ethics Journal* 3(1993): 279–86; E.J. Emanuel and N.N. Dubler, "Preserving the physician–patient relationship in the era of managed care," *JAMA* 273 (1995): 323–29; J. Balint and W. Shelton, "Regaining the initiative: Forging a new model of the patient–physician relationship," *JAMA* 275(1996): 887–91; D. Mechanic and M. Schlesinger, "The impact of managed care on patients' trust in medical care and their physicians," *JAMA* 275(1996): 1693–97.

3. Angell, "The doctor as double agent."

4. G.W. Grumet, "Health care rationing through inconvenience," *New England Journal of Medicine* 321(1989): 607–11.

5. R.F. St. Peter, M.C. Reed, P. Kemper, and D. Blumenthal, "Changes in the scope of care provided by primary care physicians," *New England Journal of Medicine* 341(1999): 1980–85.

6. R. Kuttner, "Must good HMOs go bad?" *New England Journal of Medicine* 338(1998): 1558–63, 1635–39.

7. H. Waitzkin, "Doctor–patient communication: Clinical implications of social scientific research," *JAMA* 252(1984): 2441–46; H. Waitzkin, "Information giving in medical care," *Journal of Health and Social Behavior* 26(1985): 81–101; H. Waitzkin, *The Politics of Medical Encounters: How Patients and Doctors Deal with Social Problems* (New Haven, CT: Yale University Press, 1991); D.L. Roter and J.A. Hall, *Doctors Talking with Patients/Patients Talking with Doctors* (Westport, CT: Auburn House, 1992).

8. Waitzkin, "Information giving in medical care."

9. Roter and Hall, *Doctors Talking with Patients/Patients Talking with Doctors*; M. Lipkin, S.M. Putnam, and A. Lazare, eds., *The Medical Interview: Clinical Care, Education, and Research* (New York: Springer, 1995); R.C. Smith, *The Patient's Story: Integrated Patient–Doctor Interviewing* (Boston: Little, Brown, 1996); B. Korsch and C. Harding, *Intelligent Patients' Guide to the Doctor–Patient Relationship* (New York: Oxford University Press, 1997).

10. Roter and Hall, *Doctors Talking with Patients/Patients Talking with Doctors*.

11. Waitzkin, "Doctor–patient communication"; Waitzkin, "Information giving in medical care."

12. D. Tannen, ed., *Gender and Conversational Interaction* (New York: Oxford University Press, 1993); S. Fisher, *Nursing Wounds: Nurse Practitioners, Doctors, Women Patients and the Negotiation of Meaning* (New Brunswick, NJ: Rutgers University Press, 1995).

13. R. Castillo, H. Waitzkin, Y. Villaseñor, and J.I. Escobar, "Mental health disorders and somatoform symptoms among immigrants and refugees who seek primary care services," *Archives of Family Medicine* 4(1995): 637–46.

14. R.W. Putsch, "Cross-cultural communication: The special case of interpreters in health care," *JAMA* 254(1985): 3344–48; E.J. Hardt, *The Bilingual Medical Interview* (Boston: Boston Department of Health and Hospitals and Boston Area Health Education Center, 1991); J. Sarver and D.W. Baker, "Effect of language barriers on follow-up appointments after an emergency department visit," *Journal of General Internal Medicine* 15 (2000): 256–64; K.P. Derose and D.W. Baker, "Limited English proficiency and Latinos' use of physician services," *Medical Care Research & Review* 57(2000): 76–91; D.W. Baker, R. Hayes, and J.P. Fortier, "Interpreter use and satisfaction with interpersonal aspects of care for Spanish-speaking patients," *Medical Care* 36(1998): 1461–70; R.P. Hayes and D.W. Baker, "Methodological problems in comparing English-speaking and Spanish-speaking patients' satisfaction with interpersonal aspects of care," *Medical Care* 36(1998): 230–36; D.W. Baker, R.W. Parker, M.V. Williams, W.C. Coates, and K. Pitkin, "Use and effectiveness of interpreters in an emergency department," *JAMA* 275(1996): 783–88; J.C. Hornberger, C.D. Gibson, Jr., W. Wood et al., "Eliminating language barriers for non-English-speaking patients," *Medical Care* 34(1996): 845–56; J.M. Kaufert and R.W. Putsch, "Communication through interpreters in health care: Ethical

dilemmas arising from differences in class, culture, language, and power," *Journal of Clinical Ethics* 8(1997): 71–87; D. Xuo and M.J. Fagan, "Satisfaction with methods of Spanish interpretation in an ambulatory-care clinic," *Journal of General Internal Medicine* 14(1999): 547–50; O. Carrasquillo, E.J. Orav, T.A. Brennan, and H.R. Burstin, "Impact of language barriers on patient satisfaction in an emergency department," *Journal of General Internal Medicine* 14(1999): 82–87; L.S. Morales, W.E. Cunningham, J.A. Brown, H. Liu, and R.D. Hays, "Are Latinos less satisfied with communication by health care providers?" *Journal of General Internal Medicine* 14(1999): 409–17.

15. D. Roter, M. Lipkin, Jr., and A. Korsgaard, "Sex differences in patients' and physicians' communication during primary care visits," *Medical Care* 29(1991): 1083–93.

16. Roter, Lipkin, and Korsgaard, "Sex differences"; J.A. Hall, J.A. Irish, D.L. Roter, C.M. Ehrlich, and L.H. Miller, "Satisfaction, gender, and communication in medical visits," *Medical Care* 32(1994): 1216–31; J.A. Hall, J.T. Irish, D.L. Roter, C.M. Ehrlich, and L.H. Miller, "Gender in medical encounters: An analysis of physician and patient communication in a primary-care setting," *Health Psychology* 13(1994): 384–92; D.L. Roter and J.A. Hall, "Why physician gender matters in shaping the physician–patient relationship," *Journal of Women's Health* 7(1998): 1093–97.

17. S. Woolhandler and D.U. Himmelstein, "Extreme risk: The new corporate proposition for physicians," *New England Journal of Medicine* 1995(333): 1706–8; D.R. Olmos and S. Roan, "HMO curbs prompt rising doctor protest," *Los Angeles Times* (April 14, 1996): A1.

18. American College of Physicians, *Ethics Manual*, 3rd ed. (Philadelphia: American College of Physicians, 1993); H. Brody and E. Alexander, "Gag rules and trade secrets in managed care contracts," *Archives of Internal Medicine* 157(1997): 2037–43; D.S. Feldman, D.H. Novack, and E. Gracely, "Effects of managed care on physician–patient relationships, quality of care, and the ethical practice of medicine: A physician survey," *Archives of Internal Medicine* 158(1998): 1626–32.

19. T.A. Brennan, "An ethical perspective on health care insurance reform," *American Journal of Law and Medicine* 19(1993): 37–74.

20. M.A. Rodwin, "Conflicts in managed care," *New England Journal of Medicine* 332(1995): 604–5.

21. A.C. Kao, D.C. Green, N.A. Davis, J.P. Koplan, and P.D. Cleary, "Patients' trust in their physicians: Effects of choice, continuity, and payment method," *Journal of General Internal Medicine* 13(1998): 681–86.

22. H. Waitzkin and J.D. Stoeckle, "The communication of information about illness: Clinical, sociological, and methodological considerations," *Advances in Psychosomatic Medicine* 8(1972): 180–215.

23. D.H. Novack, R. Plumer, R.L. Smith, H. Ochitill, G.R. Morrow, and J.M. Bennett, "Changes in physicians' attitudes toward telling the cancer patient," *JAMA* 241(1979): 897–900; T.R. Fried, M.D. Stein, P.S. O'Sullivan,

D.W. Brock, and D.H. Novack, "Limits of patient autonomy: Physician attitudes and practices regarding life-sustaining treatments and euthanasia," *Archives of Internal Medicine* 153(1993): 722–28.

24. T. Bodenheimer, "The HMO backlash: Righteous or reactionary?" *New England Journal of Medicine* 335(1996): 1601–4.

25. Kuttner, "Must good HMOs go bad?"

26. Olmos and Roan, "HMO curbs prompt rising doctor protest."

27. S. Sleeper, D.R. Wholey, R. Hamer, S. Schwartz, and V. Inoferio, "Trust me: Technical and institutional determinants of health maintenance organizations shifting risk to physicians," *Journal of Health and Social Behavior* 39(1998): 189–200.

28. Waitzkin, *The Politics of Medical Encounters*; H. Waitzkin, T. Britt, and C. Williams, "Narratives of aging and social problems in medical encounters with older persons," *Journal of Health and Social Behavior* 35(1994): 322–48.

## CHAPTER FIVE

1. For illustrative studies of mental health problems in primary care, see F. Lefevre, D. Reifler, P. Lee, M. Sbenghe, N. Nwadiaro, S. Verma, and P.R. Yarnold, "Screening for undetected mental disorders in high utilizers of primary care services," *Journal of General Internal Medicine* 14(1999): 425–31; E.A. Holman, R.C. Silver, and H. Waitzkin, "Prevalence and correlates of traumatic life events in immigrants and others seeking primary care," *Archives of Family Medicine* (2001, in press); F.V. DeGruy III, "Mental health diagnoses and the costs of primary care," *Journal of Family Practice* 49(2000): 311–13; K. Rost, P. Nutting, J. Smith, J.C. Coyne, L. Cooper-Patrick, and L. Rubenstein, "The role of competing demands in the treatment provided primary care patients with major depression," *Archives of Family Medicine* 9(2000): 150–54. On the extent of mental health disorders in the general population from research such as the National Comorbidity Study, see R.C. Kessler, R.L. DuPont, P. Berglund, and H.U. Wittchen, "Impairment in pure and comorbid generalized anxiety disorder and major depression at 12 months in two national surveys," *American Journal of Psychiatry* 156(1999): 1915–23; H.U. Wittchen, T.B. Ustun, and R.C. Kessler, "Diagnosing mental disorders in the community: A difference that matters?" *Psychological Medicine* 29(1999): 1021–27; R.C. Kessler, C. Barber, H.G. Birnbaum et al., "Depression in the workplace: Effects on short-term disability," *Health Affairs* 18(1999): 163–71; P.E. Greenberg, T. Sisitsky, R.C. Kessler et al., "The economic burden of anxiety disorders in the 1990s," *Journal of Clinical Psychiatry* 60(1999): 427–35; R.C. Kessler, S. Zhao, S.J. Katz et al., "Past-year use of outpatient services for psychiatric problems in the National Comorbidity Survey," *American Journal of Psychiatry* 156(1999): 115–23; R.C. Kessler, G. Borges, and E.E. Walters, "Prevalence of and risk factors for life-

time suicide attempts in the National Comorbidity Survey," *Archives of General Psychiatry* 56(1999): 617–26.

2. National initiatives that focus on mental health in the primary care sector include those of the National Institute of Mental Health (details at <www.nih.nimh.gov>), the Agency for Healthcare Research and Quality (<www.ahrq.gov>), and the Robert Wood Johnson Foundation (<www.rwjf.org>). For examples of local interventions, see K. Rost, P.A. Nutting, J. Smith, and J.J. Werner, "Designing and implementing a primary care intervention trial to improve the quality and outcome of care for major depression," *General Hospital Psychiatry* 22(2000): 66–77; W.W. Williams, Jr., K. Rost, A.J. Dietrich et al., "Primary care physicians' approach to depressive disorders: Effects of physician specialty and practice structure," *Archives of Family Medicine* 8(1999): 58–67.

3. R. Castillo, H. Waitzkin, Y. Villaseñor, and J.I. Escobar, "Mental health disorders and somatoform symptoms among immigrants and refugees who seek primary care services," *Archives of Family Medicine* 4(1995): 637–46.

4. See note 14 for chapter 4.

5. G.N. Hoang and R.V. Erickson, "Guidelines for providing medical care to Southeast Asian refugees," *JAMA* 248(1982): 710–14; J.D. Mull and D.S. Mull, "A visit with a curandero," *Western Journal of Medicine* 139 (1983): 730–36; D. Nguyen, "Culture shock: A review of Vietnamese culture and its concepts of health and disease," *Western Journal of Medicine* 142(1985): 409–12; D. Eisenberg, R. Kessler, C. Foster et al., "Unconventional medicine in the United States: Prevalence, costs, and patterns of use," *New England Journal of Medicine* 328(1993): 246–52; D.M. Eisenberg, R.B. Davis, S.L. Ettner et al., "Trends in alternative medicine use in the United States, 1990–1997: Results of a follow-up national survey," *JAMA* 280(1998): 1569–75.

6. A. Kleinman, *The Illness Narratives* (New York: Basic Books, 1988); A. Kleinman and A.E. Becker, "'Sociosomatics': The contributions of anthropology to psychosomatic medicine," *Psychosomatic Medicine* 60(1998): 389–93; J. Rubel, C.W. O'Nell, and R. Collado-Ardón, *Susto: A Folk Illness* (Berkeley: University of California Press, 1984).

7. H. Waitzkin, *The Politics of Medical Encounters: How Patients and Doctors Deal with Social Problems* (New Haven, CT: Yale University Press, 1991).

8. J.I. Escobar, "Cross-cultural aspects of the somatization trait," *Hospital and Community Psychiatry* 38(1987): 174–80; J.I. Escobar, H. Waitzkin, R.C. Silver, M. Gara, and A. Holman, "Abridged somatization: A study in primary care," *Psychosomatic Medicine* 60(1998): 466–72; Holman, Silver, and Waitzkin, "Prevalence and correlates of traumatic life events"; J. Coreil and J.D. Mull, eds., *Anthropology and Primary Health Care* (Boulder, CO: Westview, 1990).

9. N. Sartorius, "Refugee mental health: Issues and problems," in H.-T.

Lo and E. Yeh, eds., *Critical Condition: Refugee Mental Health* (Toronto: Hong Fook Mental Health Association, 1992). Sartorius presents the definitions used by the World Health Organization and affiliated organizations: "The definition of the word *refugee* as '. . . a person who owing to well-founded fear of being persecuted for reasons of race, religion, nationality, [or] membership in a particular group of political opinion is outside the country of his nationality' served to define the role of the United Nations High Commission for Refugees. It was subsequently amended—for example, by the Organization of African Unity, which added that 'persons fleeing from war, civil disturbance, and violence of any kind' should also be considered refugees. Subsequently, the definition was even further amended to include persons fleeing from extreme economic hardship as well as persons displaced within the borders of their own country (provided that they met the other requirement of being in vital danger unless they left their usual abode)."

10. U.S. Code (Annotated), *Title 8, Aliens and Nationality* (Dayton, OH: Lexis Law Publishing, 2000), 8 USCS § 1101. The U.S. Code (Annotated) defines *refugee* and specifies the discretion of the administrative branch of government as follows: "The term 'refugee' means (A) any person who is outside any country of such person's nationality or, in the case of a person having no nationality, is outside any country in which such person last habitually resided, and who is unable or unwilling to return to, and is unable or unwilling to avail himself or herself of the protection of, that country because of persecution or a well-founded fear of persecution on account of race, religion, nationality, membership in a particular social group, or political opinion, or (B) in such special circumstances as the President after appropriate consultation (as defined in section 207(e) of this Act [8 USCS § 1157(e)]) may specify, any person who is within the country of such person's nationality or, in the case of a person having no nationality, within the country in which such person is habitually residing, and who is persecuted or who has a well-founded fear of persecution on account of race, religion, nationality, membership in a particular social group, or political opinion. The term 'refugee' does not include any person who ordered, incited, assisted, or otherwise participated in the persecution of any person on account of race, religion, nationality, membership in a particular social group, or political opinion. For purposes of determinations under this Act, a person who has been forced to abort a pregnancy or to undergo involuntary sterilization, or who has been persecuted for failure or refusal to undergo such a procedure or for other resistance to a coercive population control program, shall be deemed to have been persecuted on account of political opinion, and a person who has a wellfounded fear that he or she will be forced to undergo such a procedure or subject to persecution for such failure, refusal, or resistance shall be deemed to have a well-founded fear of persecution on account of political opinion."

11. U.S. Bureau of the Census, *1980 Census of the Population* (Washing-

ton, DC: U.S. Department of Commerce [Publication PC 80-1-C1], 1983); U.S. Bureau of the Census, *1990 Census of the Population* (Van Nuys, CA: Bureau of the Census, 1992).

12. A. Aron, "Applications of psychology to the assessment of refugees seeking political asylum," *Applied Psychology* 41(1992): 77–91.

13. C.R. Cervantes, V.N. Salgado de Snyder, and A.M. Padilla, "Post-traumatic stress disorder in immigrants from Central America and Mexico," *Hospital and Community Psychiatry* 40(1989): 615–19.

14. M. Eisenbruch, "From post-traumatic stress disorder to cultural bereavement: Diagnosis of Southeast Asian refugees," *Social Science & Medicine* 33(1991): 673–80; R.F. Mollica, Y. Caspi-Yavin, P. Bollini et al., "The Harvard Trauma Questionnaire: Validating a cross-cultural instrument for measuring torture, trauma, and posttraumatic stress disorder in Indochinese refugees," *Journal of Nervous and Mental Diseases* 180(1992): 111–16; S.I. Hsu, "Somatisation among Asian refugees and immigrants as a culturally-shaped illness behaviour," *Annals of the Academy of Medicine of Singapore* 28(1999): 841–45; T. O'Hare and T. Van Tran, "Substance abuse among Southeast Asians in the U.S.: Implications for practice and research," *Social Work in Health Care* 26(1998): 69–80.

15. E.H.B. Lin, W.B. Carter, and A.M. Kleinman, "An exploration of somatization among Asian refugees and immigrants in primary care," *American Journal of Public Health* 75(1985): 1080–84; L.J. Moore and J. Boehnlein, "Posttraumatic stress disorder, depression, and somatic symptoms in U.S. Mien patients," *Journal of Nervous and Mental Diseases* 179 (1991): 728–33; R.F. Mollica, K. Donelan, S. Tor et al., "The effect of trauma and confinement on functional health and mental health status of Cambodians living in Thailand–Cambodia border camps," *JAMA* 270(1993): 581–86; R.F. Mollica, "Waging a new kind of war: Invisible wounds," *Scientific American* 282(2000): 54–57; R.F. Mollica, K. McInnes, C. Poole, and S. Tor, "Dose-effect relationships of trauma to symptoms of depression and post-traumatic stress disorder among Cambodian survivors of mass violence," *British Journal of Psychiatry* 173(1998): 482–88; R.F. Mollica, K. McInnes, T. Pham et al., "The dose-effect relationships between torture and psychiatric symptoms in Vietnamese ex-political detainees and a comparison group," *Journal of Nervous & Mental Disease* 186(1998): 543–53.

16. B. Brodsky, "Mental health attitudes and practices of Soviet Jewish immigrants," *Health and Social Work* 13(1988): 130–36; R. Kohn, J. Flaherty, and I. Levav, "Mental health attitudes and practices of Soviet immigrants," *Israel Journal of Psychiatry* 27(1990): 131–44.

17. W. Katon, A.M. Kleinman, and G. Rosen, "Depression and somatization: A review," *American Journal of Medicine* 72(1982): 127–35; W. Katon, R. Ries, and A. Kleinman, "The prevalence of somatization in primary care," *Comprehensive Psychiatry* 25(1984): 208–15.

18. C. Kaplan, M. Lipkin, and G.H. Gordon, "Somatization in primary care," *Journal of General Internal Medicine* 3(1988): 177–90.

19. G.R. Smith, Jr., *Somatization Disorder in the Medical Setting* (Washington, DC: U.S. Government Printing Office, National Institute of Mental Health [DHHS Pub. No. (ADM) 90-1631], 1990).

20. American Psychiatric Association, *Diagnostic and Statistical Manual of Mental Disorders. DSM-IV*, 4th ed. (Washington, DC: American Psychiatric Association, 1994).

21. E. Shorter, *From Paralysis to Fatigue: A History of Psychosomatic Illness in the Modern Era* (New York: Free Press, 1992).

22. American Psychiatric Association, *Diagnostic and Statistical Manual of Mental Disorders*, 445–69.

23. I.K. Zola, "Culture and symptoms: An analysis of patients' presenting complaints," *American Sociological Review* 31(1966): 615–30.

24. K.L. Pliskin, *Silent Boundaries: Cultural Constraints on Sickness and Diagnosis of Iranians in Israel* (New Haven, CT: Yale University Press, 1987).

25. Lin, Carter, and Kleinman, "Exploration of somatization."

26. R. Angel and P.J. Guarnaccia, "Mind, body, and culture: Somatization among Hispanics," *Social Science & Medicine* 28(1989): 1229–38.

27. G.R. Smith, Jr., R.A. Monson, and D.C. Ray, "Patients with multiple unexplained symptoms: Their characteristics, functional health, and health care utilization," *Archives of Internal Medicine* 146(1986): 69–72.

28. Smith, Monson, and Ray, "Patients with multiple unexplained symptoms"; DeGruy, "Mental health diagnoses and the costs of primary care."

29. Castillo, Waitzkin, Escobar, and Villaseñor, "Mental health disorders and somatoform symptoms."

30. Hoang and Erickson, "Guidelines for providing medical care to Southeast Asian refugees"; Mollica, Caspi-Yavin, Bollini et al., "The Harvard Trauma Questionnaire."

31. Angel and Guarnaccia, "Mind, body, and culture"; J.I. Escobar, G. Canino, M. Rubio-Stipec, and M. Bravo, "Somatic symptoms after a natural disaster: A prospective study," *American Journal of Psychiatry* 148(1992): 965–67.

32. E. Shorter, *From the Mind into the Body: The Cultural Origins of Psychosomatic Symptoms* (New York: Free Press, 1994).

## CHAPTER SIX

1. A.L. Kellermann and B.B. Hackman, "Emergency department patient dumping: An analysis of interhospital transfers to the regional medical center at Memphis, Tennessee," *American Journal of Public Health* 78(1988): 1287–92; R.L. Schiff, D.A. Ansell, J.E. Schlosser et al., "Transfers to a public hospital: A prospective study of 467 patients," *New England Journal of Medicine* 314(1986): 552–57; W.G. Reed, K.A. Cawley, and R.J. Anderson, "The effect of a public hospital's transfer policy on patient care," *New England Journal of Medicine* 22(1986): 1428–32; W.W. Bera,

"Preventing 'patient dumping': The Supreme Court turns away the sixth circuit's interpretation of EMTALA," *Houston Law Review* 36(1999): 615.

2. E.R. Brown, R. Burciaga Valdez, H. Morgenstern, T. Bradley, and C. Hafner, *Californians Without Health Insurance: A Report to the California Legislature* (Berkeley: California Policy Seminar, University of California, 1987); E.R. Brown and M.R. Cousinau, *Assessing Indigent Health Care Needs and Use of County Health Services* (Berkeley: California Policy Seminar, University of California, 1987); H. Waitzkin and F.A. Hubbell, "Truth's search for power: Critical applications to community-oriented primary care and small-area analysis," *Medical Care Review* 49(1992): 161–89; D.J. Reese, R.E. Ahern, S. Nair, J.D. O'Faire, and C. Warren, "Hospice access and use by African Americans: Addressing cultural and institutional barriers through participatory action research," *Social Work* 44(1999): 549–59; H. Grason, B. Aliza, V.L. Hutchins, B. Guyer, and C. Minkovitz, "Pediatrician-led community child health initiatives: Case summaries from the evaluation of the community access to child health program," *Pediatrics* 103(1999): 1394–419.

3. P. Braveman, G. Oliva, M.G. Miller, R. Reiter, and S. Egerter, "Adverse outcomes and lack of health insurance in an eight-county area of California, 1982 to 1986," *New England Journal of Medicine* 321(1989): 508–13; J.S. Mandelblatt, R.S. Adler, N.M. Bennett et al., "Divisions of general medicine: Ambulatory care activities and responses to cost containment," *Journal of General Internal Medicine* 2(1987): 388–93; J. Gates-Williams, S. Schear, and M. Tervalon, "Health-care administration and the county hospital: Community activism as a catalyst for change," *Journal of Health and Human Resources Admininstration* 10(1988): 297–310; N.A. Jewell and K.M. Russell, "Increasing access to prenatal care: An evaluation of minority health coalitions' early pregnancy project," *Journal of Community Health Nursing* 17(2000): 93–105.

4. These estimates are based on 1990 census data, the latest available at the time of this writing; see <http://sun3.lib.uci.edu/~dtsang/ocinc.htm> (September 2000).

5. County Housing Market Trends, September 2000 <http://www.quick.net/lfc/trends/ochsng.html>.

6. For further details on these publications concerning local-access problems, see chapter 2 and Waitzkin and Hubbell, "Truth's search for power." An overview of the early phases of this local advocacy work appeared in V. Mayster, H. Waitzkin, F.A. Hubbell, and L. Rucker, "Local advocacy for the medically indigent: Strategies and accomplishments in one county," *JAMA* 263(1990): 262–68.

7. B.V. Akin, L. Rucker, F.A. Hubbell, R.C. Cygan, and H. Waitzkin, "Access to medical care in a medically indigent population," *Journal of General Internal Medicine* 4(1989): 216–20.

8. F.A. Hubbell, H. Waitzkin, L. Rucker, B.V. Akin, and M.G. Heide, "Financial barriers to medical care: A prospective study in a university-

affiliated community clinic," *American Journal of Medical Sciences* 297(1989): 158–62.

9. F.A. Hubbell, H. Waitzkin, S.I. Mishra, and J. Dombrink, "Evaluating health-care needs of the poor: A community-oriented approach," *American Journal of Medicine* 87(1989): 127–31; F.A. Hubbell, H. Waitzkin, S.I. Mishra, J. Dombrink, and L.R. Chávez, "Access to medical care for documented and undocumented Latinos in a southern California county," *Western Journal of Medicine* 154(1991): 414–17.

10. N. Rimsha, H. Waitzkin, I. Peña et al., "Local research and legal advocacy for the medically indigent," *American Journal of Public Health* 86(1996): 883–85.

11. For perspectives on the issue of corporate management in the context of academic medical centers, see E. Ginzberg, H.S. Berliner, and M. Ostow, *Changing U.S. Health Care: A Study of Four Metropolitan Areas* (Boulder, CO: Westview, 1993); J.C. Robinson, "Capital finance and ownership conversions in health care," *Health Affairs* 19(2000): 56–71; F.W. Hafferty, "Managed medical education?" *Academic Medicine* 74(1999): 972–79; J.D. Stoeckle, "The market pushes education from ward to office, from acute to chronic illness and prevention: Will case-method teaching-learning change?" *Archives of Internal Medicine* 160(2000): 273–80.

12. The early history of this process appears in H. Waitzkin, B.V. Akin, L.M. de la Maza et al., "Deciding against corporate management of a state-supported academic medical center," *New England Journal of Medicine* 315(1986): 1299–1304.

## CHAPTER SEVEN

1. H. Waitzkin, "Why it's time for a national health program in the United States," *Western Journal of Medicine* 150(1989): 101–7; J.S. Hacker and T. Skocpol, "The new politics of U.S. health policy," *Journal of Health Politics, Policy & Law* 22(1997): 315–38; V. Navarro, *The Politics of Health Policy: The U.S. Reforms, 1980–1994* (Cambridge, MA: Blackwell, 1994); T. Skocpol, *Boomerang: Clinton's Health Security Effort and the Turn Against Government in U.S. Politics* (New York: Norton, 1996).

2. R.J. Blendon, J.M. Benson, M. Brodie et al., "Voters and health care in the 1996 election," *JAMA* 277(1997): 1253–58; R.J. Blendon, J.M. Benson, M. Brodie et al., "Voters and health care in the 1998 election," *JAMA* 282 (1999): 189–94; K. Donelan, R.J. Blendon, C. Schoen, K. Davis, and K. Binns, "The cost of health system change: Public discontent in five nations," *Health Affairs* 18(1999): 206–16.

3. D.U. Himmelstein, S. Woolhandler, and the Writing Committee of the Working Group on Program Design, Physicians for a National Health Program, "A national health program for the United States: A physicians' proposal," *New England Journal of Medicine* 320(1989): 102–8.

4. Committee on the Costs of Medical Care, *Medical Care for the American People: The Final Report of the Committee on the Costs of Medical Care* (adopted October 31, 1932) (New York: Arno Press, 1972).

5. B. Stuart and C. Zacker, "Who bears the burden of Medicaid drug copayment policies?" *Health Affairs* 18(1999): 201–12; see also H.M. Leichter, "The poor and managed care in the Oregon experience," *Journal of Health Politics, Policy & Law* 24(1999): 1173–84; J.E. Ware, Jr., R.J. Brook, W.H. Rogers et al., "Comparison of health outcomes at a health maintenance organization with those of fee-for-service care," *Lancet* 1(1986): 1017–22; J.E. Ware, Jr., M.S. Bayliss, W.H. Rogers et al., "Differences in 4-year health outcomes for elderly and poor, chronically ill patients treated in HMO and fee-for-service systems," *JAMA* 276(1996): 1039–47.

6. R.G. Evans, M.L. Barer, and C. Hertzman, "The twenty-year experiment: Accounting for, explaining, and evaluating health care cost-containment in Canada and the United States," *Annual Review of Public Health* 12(1991): 481–518; R. Evans and N.P. Roos, "What is right about the Canadian health-care system?" *Milbank Quarterly* 77(1999): 393–99; K. Wilson, "Health care, federalism and the new social union," *CMAJ* 162(2000): 1171–74; D. Coburn, "Phases of capitalism, welfare states, medical dominance, and health care in Ontario," *International Journal of Health Services* 29(1999): 833–51.

7. U.S. General Accounting Office, *Canadian Health Insurance: Lessons for the United States* (Washington, DC: Government Printing Office [GAO Publ. No. GAO/HRD-91-90; B-244081], 1991).

8. Waitzkin, "Why it's time for a national health program."

9. A.C. Enthoven, *Theory and Practice of Managed Competition in Health Care Finance* (Amsterdam: North-Holland, 1988), 65–67.

10. A.C. Enthoven, "Consumer-choice health plan," *New England Journal of Medicine* 298(1978): 650–58, 709–20.

11. A.C. Enthoven, *Health Plan: The Only Practical Solution to the Soaring Cost of Medical Care* (Reading, MA: Addison-Wesley, 1980).

12. H. Waitzkin, "The strange career of managed competition: Military failure to medical success?" *American Journal of Public Health* 84 (1994): 482–89.

13. A.C. Enthoven, "Managed competition in health care and the unfinished agenda," *Health Care Finance Review Suppl.* (1986): 105–19.

14. A.C. Enthoven and R. Kronick, "A consumer-choice health plan for the 1990's," *New England Journal of Medicine* 320(1989): 29–37, 94–101.

15. Bruce Shapiro, "Zoe Baird," *Los Angeles Times* (January 7, 1993): B11; *Lancet*, "U.S. health reforms: Clichés, cost, and Mrs. C.," *Lancet* 341(1993): 791–92.

16. P. Ellwood, A.C. Enthoven, and L. Etheredge, "The Jackson Hole initiatives for a twenty-first century American health care system," *Health Economics* 1(1992): 149–68.

17. E.R. Brown, "Health USA: A national health program for the United States," *JAMA* 267(1992): 552–58; J. Garamendi, *California Health Care in the 21st Century: A Vision for Reform* (Sacramento: California Department of Insurance, 1992); P. Starr, *The Logic of Healthcare Reform* (Knoxville, TN: Whittle Direct Books, 1992); P. Starr and W.A. Zelman, "A bridge to compromise: Competition under a budget," *Health Affairs* (Millwood) 12 suppl. (1993): 7–23.

18. J.P. Hadley and K. Langwell, "Managed care in the United States: Promises, evidence to date and future directions," *Health Policy* 19(1991): 91–118; J.K. Iglehart, "Managed competition," *New England Journal of Medicine* 328(1993): 1208–12; R. Kronick, D.C. Goodman, J. Wennberg, and E. Wagner, "The marketplace in health care reform: The demographic limitations of managed competition," *New England Journal of Medicine* 328 (1993): 148–52.

19. For studies of administrative costs, see note 5 of chapter 1. When limited managed care principles were introduced into the British National Health Service, administrative costs rose from 8 to 11 percent between 1995 and 1996, and clerical staff increased by 15 percent: J. LeGrand, "Competition, cooperation, or control?: Tales from the British National Health Service," *Health Affairs* 18(May–June 1999): 27–39. Other pertinent studies of managed care and its implications for a national health program appear in the following special issue: *Journal of Health Politics, Policy & Law* 24(October 1999).

20. W.A. Glaser, "The competition vogue and its outcomes," *Lancet* 341(1993): 805–12; *Lancet*, "U.S. health reforms."

21. R.J. Blendon, M. Brodie, and J. Benson, "What happened to Americans' support for the Clinton health plan?" *Health Affairs* 14(1995): 7–23; R.J. Blendon, M. Brodie, T.S. Hyams, and J.M. Benson, "The American public and the critical choices for health system reform," *JAMA* 271(1994): 1539–44; R.J. Blendon, T.S. Hyams, and J.M. Benson, "Bridging the gap between expert and public views on health care reform," *JAMA* 269(1993): 2573–78.

22. U.S. General Accounting Office, *Canadian Health Insurance*; T.R. Marmor, "Commentary on Canadian health insurance: Lessons for the United States," *International Journal of Health Services* 23(1993): 45–62.

23. Shapiro, "Zoe Baird"; *Lancet*, "U.S. health reforms."

24. A.C. Enthoven, "Choosing strategies and selecting weapon systems" (address before Naval War College, Newport, RI, June 6, 1963), in Samuel A. Tucker, ed., *A Modern Design for Defense Decision: A McNamara–Hitch–Enthoven Anthology* (Washington, DC: Industrial College of the Armed Forces, 1966).

25. Waitzkin, "The strange career of managed competition."

26. W. Berry, *What Are People For?* (San Francisco: North Point Press, 1990), 135.

27. Himmelstein, Woolhandler, and the Writing Committee of the

Working Group on Program Design, "A national health program for the United States"; K. Grumbach, T. Bodenheimer, D.U. Himmelstein, and S. Woolhandler, "Liberal benefits, conversative spending: The Physicians for a National Health Program proposal," *JAMA* 265(1991): 2549–54; C. Harrington, C. Cassel, C.L. Estes et al., "A national long-term care program for the United States: A caring vision," *JAMA* 266(1991): 3023–29.

28. Navarro, *The Politics of Health Policy*.

29. Grumbach et al., "Liberal benefits, conversative spending."

30. Congressional Budget Office, *An Analysis of the Managed Competition Act* (Washington, DC: Government Printing Office, 1994); "H.R. 3222, the Managed Competition Act of 1993," hearing before the Committee on Education and Labor, House of Representatives, 103rd Congress (Washington, DC, March 3, 1994); "Health care cost control and managed competition," hearing of the Senate Finance Committee, 103rd Congress (Washington, DC, May 4, 1994); "Overview and estimated revenue effects of the Managed Competition Act of 1993 (H.R. 3222 and S. 1579)," hearing of the Joint Committee on Taxation, 103rd Congress (Washington, DC, May 6, 1994).

## CHAPTER EIGHT

1. For research on social class differences in health outcomes, see note 46 of chapter 3, as well as V. Navarro, "A historical review (1965–1997) of studies on class, health, and quality of life: A personal account," *International Journal of Health Services* 28(1998): 389–406; and "The widening gap in death rates among income groups in the United States from 1967 to 1986," *International Journal of Health Services* 30(2000): 13–26.

2. P.M. Lantz et al., "Socioeconomic factors, health behaviors, and mortality: Results from a nationally representative prospective study of U.S. adults," *JAMA* 279(1998): 1703–8.

3. For research on racial differences in health outcomes, and on the interactions among race, social class, and gender, see notes 50–57 of chapter 3. For McKinley County, New Mexico, see U.S. Department of Health and Human Services, Health Resources and Services Administration, Community Health Status Indicators Project, September 2000 (<http://www.communityhealth.hrsa.gov/countyinfo.asp>).

4. For further research on the impacts of race versus class, see L.E. Montgomery, J.L. Kiely, and G. Pappas, "The effects of poverty, race, and family structure on U.S. children's health: Data from the NHIS, 1978 through 1980 and 1989 through 1991," *American Journal of Public Health* 86(1996): 1401–5; N. Krieger and S. Sidney, "Racial discrimination and blood pressure: The CARDIA Study of young black and white adults," *American Journal of Public Health* 86(1996): 1370–78.

5. A.L. Rosenbloom, D.V. House, and W.E. Winter, "Noninsulin dependent diabetes mellitus (NIDDM) in minority youth: Research priori-

ties and needs," *Clinical Pediatrics* 37(1998): 143–52; J.A. Griffin, S.S. Gilliland, G. Pérez, D. Helitzer, and J.S. Carter, "Participant satisfaction with a culturally appropriate diabetes education program: The Native American Diabetes Project," *Diabetes Educator* 25(1999): 351–63.

6. Navarro, "A historical review."

7. See notes 51, 52, and 53 of chapter 3.

8. See notes 55 and 56 of chapter 3.

9. See note 59 of chapter 3.

10. See note 58 of chapter 3.

11. R. Karasek and T. Theorell, *Healthy Work: Stress, Productivity, and the Reconstruction of Working Life* (New York: Basic Books, 1990); R. Karasek, "Labour participation and work quality policy: Outline of an alternative economic vision," *WHO Regional Publications. European Series* 81(1999): 169–239; K. Steenland, L. Fine, K. Belkic et al., "Research findings linking workplace factors to CVD outcomes," *Occupational Medicine* 15(2000): 7–68.

12. S. Allende, *La Realidad Médico-Social Chilena* (Santiago: Ministerio de Salubridad, Previsión y Asistencia Social, 1939).

13. H. Waitzkin, *The Second Sickness: Contradictions of Capitalist Health Care* (Lanham, MD: Rowman & Littlefield, 2000), 189–207.

14. C.W. Mills, *The Sociological Imagination* (New York: Grove, 1959), 8–11.

15. F.F. Piven and R.A. Cloward, *Regulating the Poor* (New York: Vintage, 1993), and *The Breaking of the American Social Compact* (New York: New Press, 1998).

16. A. Gorz, *Socialism and Revolution* (Garden City, NY: Anchor, 1973), and *Capitalism, Socialism, Ecology* (London: Verso, 1994).

17. P. Buhle, *From the Knights of Labor to the New World Order: Essays on Labor and Culture* (New York: Garland, 1997), and *Taking Care of Business: Samuel Gompers, George Meany, Lane Kirkland, and the Tragedy of American Labor* (New York: Monthly Review Press, 1999).

18. S.A. Magnus and S.S. Mick, "Medical schools, affirmative action, and the neglected role of social class," *American Journal of Public Health* 90(2000): 1197–1201; K. DeVille, "Defending diversity: Affirmative action and medical education," *American Journal of Public Health* 89(1999): 1256–61; G. Strayhorn, "Preadmissions programs and enrollment of underrepresented minority students before and during successful challenges to affirmative action," *Journal of the National Medical Association* 91(1999): 350–56.

19. M. Goldstein, *Alternative Health Care: Medicine, Miracle, or Mirage?* (Philadelphia: Temple University Press, 1999).

20. K. Stocker, H. Waitzkin, and C. Iriart, "The exportation of managed care to Latin America," *New England Journal of Medicine* 340(1999): 1131–36; C. Iriart, E. Merhy, and H. Waitzkin, "Managed care in Latin America: The new common sense in health policy reform," *Social Science & Medicine* (2001, in press); H. Waitzkin and C. Iriart, "How the United States exports

managed care to Third World countries," *Monthly Review* 52(May 2000): 21–35; M. Rao, ed., *Disinvesting in Health: The World Bank's Prescriptions for Health* (New Delhi: Sage, 1999); M. Turshen, *Privatizing Health Services in Africa* (New Brunswick, NJ: Rutgers University Press, 1999).

21. H. Hu, E. Chivian, A. Haines, and M. McCally, eds., *Critical Condition: Human Health and the Environment: A Report by Physicians for Social Responsibility* (Cambridge, MA: MIT Press, 1993); A.J. McMichael, ed., *Climate Change and Human Health: An Assessment Prepared by a Task Group on Behalf of WHO, WMO & UNEP* (Geneva: World Health Organization, 1996).

## CHAPTER NINE

1. E.G. Mishler, J.A. Clark, J. Ingelfinger, and M.P. Simon, "The language of attentive patient care: A comparison of two medical interviews," *Journal of General Internal Medicine* 4(1989): 325–35; H. Waitzkin, *The Politics of Medical Encounters: How Patients and Doctors Deal with Social Problems* (New Haven, CT: Yale University Press, 1991).

2. Mishler, Clark, Ingelfinger, and Simon, "The language of attentive patient care"; R.C. Smith, *The Patient's Story* (Boston: Little, Brown, 1996).

3. For example, D.B. Reuben, G. Wolde-Tsadik, B. Pardamean et al., "The use of targeting criteria in hospitalized HMO patients: Results from the demonstration phase of the Hospitalized Older Persons Evaluation (HOPE) Study," *Journal of the American Geriatrics Society* 40(1992): 482–88.

4. V. Brezinka and F. Kittel, "Psychosocial factors of coronary heart disease in women: A review," *Social Science & Medicine* 42(1996): 1351–65.

5. Cf. D.L. Roter and J.A. Hall, *Doctors Talking with Patients/Patients Talking with Doctors* (Westport, CT: Auburn House, 1992).

6. R.D. Laing and A. Esterson, *Sanity, Madness and the Family* (Baltimore: Penguin, 1970); T.A. Kupers, *Public Therapy* (New York: Free Press, 1981); K. Davis, "The process of problem (re)formulation in psychotherapy," *Sociology of Health and Illness* 8(1986): 44–74; K. Davis, *Power Under the Microscope: Toward a Grounded Theory of Gender Relations in Medical Encounters* (Dortrecht, Holland: Foris, 1988).

7. Depression Guideline Panel, *Depression in Primary Care* (Rockville, MD: Agency for Health Care Policy and Research [AHCPR Publication No. 93-0550], 1993) (<http://text.nlm.nih.gov/ftrs/tocview>).

8. H. Waitzkin, T. Britt, and C. Williams, "Narratives of aging and social problems in medical encounters with older persons," *Journal of Health and Social Behavior* 35(1994): 322–48.

9. H. Waitzkin and T. Britt, "Changing the structure of medical discourse: Implications of cross-national comparisons," *Journal of Health and Social Behavior* 30(1989): 436–49; H. Waitzkin, *The Politics of Medical Encounters: How Patients and Doctors Deal with Social Problems* (New Haven, CT: Yale University Press, 1991), chapter 11.

10. D.U. Himmelstein, S. Woolhandler, and the Writing Committee of

the Working Group on Program Design, Physicians for a National Health Program, "A national health program for the United States: A physicians' proposal," *New England Journal of Medicine* 320(1989): 102–8; K. Grumbach, T. Bodenheimer, D.U. Himmelstein, and S. Woolhandler, "Liberal benefits, conversative spending: The Physicians for a National Health Program proposal," *JAMA* 265(1991): 2549–54; C. Harrington, C. Cassel, C.L. Estes et al., "A national long-term care program for the United States: A caring vision," *JAMA* 266(1991): 3023–29; G.D. Schiff, A.B. Bindman, and T.A. Brennan, "A better-quality alternative: Single-payer national health system reform," *JAMA* 272(1994): 803–8.

11. S. Woolhandler and D.U. Himmelstein, "Extreme risk: The new corporate proposition for physicians," *New England Journal of Medicine* 333(1995): 1706–8.

12. For analyses of administrative costs, see note 5 of chapter 1.

13. U.S. General Accounting Office, *Canadian Health Insurance: Lessons for the United States* (Washington, DC: Government Printing Office, 1991).

14. K.M. Langwell, V.S. Staines, and N. Gordon, *The Effects of Managed Care on Use and Costs of Health Services* (Washington, DC: Congressional Budget Office, 1992); J.R. Gabel and T. Rice, "Is managed competition a field of dreams?" *Journal of American Health Policy* 3(1993): 19–24; H. Waitzkin, "The strange career of managed competition: From military failure to medical success?" *American Journal of Public Health* 84(1994): 482–89.

15. See note 5 of chapter 1.

16. For a classic analysis of the magnitude of excessive clinical activities by physicians, see note 18 of chapter 2.

17. S. Asch, "Does fear of immigration authorities deter tuberculosis patients from seeking care?" *Western Journal of Medicine* 161(1994): 373–76; F.A. Hubbell, H. Waitzkin, S.I. Mishra, J. Dombrink, and L.R. Chavez, "Access to medical care for documented and undocumented Latinos in a southern California county," *Western Journal of Medicine* 154(1991): 414–17; C.J. Gonsalves, "The psychological effects of political repression on Chilean exiles in the U.S.," *American Journal of Orthopsychiatry* 60(1990): 143–53.

18. R.F. Mollica, G. Wyshak, J. Lavelle et al., "Assessing symptom change in Southeast Asian refugee survivors of mass violence and torture," *American Journal of Psychiatry* 147(1990): 83–88; P. Morris and D. Silove, "Cultural influences in psychotherapy with refugee survivors of torture and trauma," *Hospital and Community Psychiatry* 43(1992): 820–24; H. Waitzkin and H. Magaña, "The black box in somatization: Narrative, culture, and unexplained physical symptoms," *Social Science & Medicine* 45(1997): 811–25.

19. J.L Herman, *Trauma and Recovery* (New York: Basic Books, 1992).

20. J.W. Pennebaker, "Confession, inhibition, and disease," *Advances in Experimental Social Psychology* 22(1989): 211–44; J.W. Pennebaker, "Putting stress into words: Health, linguistic, and therapeutic implications," *Behavioral Research and Therapeutics* 31(1993): 539–49; J.W. Pennebaker and

J.D. Seagal, "Special section: Narrative in psychotherapy: The emerging metaphor—forming a story: The health benefits of narrative," *Journal of Clinical Psychology* 10(1999): 1243–55; J.M. Richards, W.E. Beal, J.D. Seagal, and J.W. Pennebaker, "Effects of disclosure of traumatic events on illness behavior among psychiatric prison inmates," *Journal of Abnormal Psychology* 109(2000): 156–61.

21. P. Freire, *Pedagogy of the Oppressed* (New York: Herder & Herder, 1970); *Pedagogy of Hope* (New York: Continuum, 1994); *Pedagogy of Freedom: Ethics, Democracy, and Civic Courage* (Lanham, MD: Rowman & Littlefield, 1998).

22. J.R. Magaña, J.B. Ferreira-Pinto, M. Blair, and A. Mata, "Una pedagogia de concientización para la prevención del VIH/SIDA," *Revista Latino Americana de Psicología* 24(1–2) (1992): 97–108; N. Wallerstein and E. Bernstein, "Empowerment education: Freire's ideas adapted to health education," *Health Education Quarterly* 15(1988): 379–94; N. Wallerstein, "Powerlessness, empowerment, and health: Implications for health promotion programs," *American Journal of Health Promotion* 6(1992): 197–205; N. Wallerstein, V. Sánchez-Merki, and L. Dow, "Freirian praxis in health education and community organizing: A case study of an adolescent prevention program," in M. Minkler, ed., *Community Organizing and Community Building for Health* (London: Routledge, 1997).

23. R. Mollica, "The trauma story: The psychiatric care of refugee survivors of violence and torture," in F. Ochberg, ed., *Post-Traumatic Therapy and Victims of Violence* (New York: Brunner/Mazel, 1988), 295–314; Herman, *Trauma and Recovery*.

24. M. Minkler and N. Wallerstein, "Improving health through community organizing and community building," in M. Minkler, ed., *Community Organizing and Community Building for Health* (London: Routledge, 1997).

25. C. Odets, *Waiting for Lefty* (New York: Grove Press, 1993 [1935]), 25–29.

# index

◆ ◆

### About the Author

**HOWARD WAITZKIN** is professor and director at the Division of Community Medicine, Department of Family and Community Medicine, University of New Mexico. Since receiving his doctorate in sociology and a degree in medicine from Harvard University, he has worked with several community-based health projects and has written numerous articles and books on health policy, community medicine, and patient–doctor communication, including *The Politics of Medical Encounters: How Patients and Doctors Deal with Social Problems* (1991) and *The Second Sickness: Contradictions of Capitalist Health Care* (Rowman & Littlefield, 2000).